Advance Praise for
The Game On! Diet

"Reading *Game On!* is like spending a day in the writer's room with Krista Vernoff—funny, candid, foulmouthed good time."
—Shonda Rhimes, creator of *Grey's Anatomy*

"*The Game On! Diet* is a smart and balanced health and fitness plan in a fun, competitive, and highly motivating format. It doesn't get much better than that!"
—Dr. Zoanne Clack, writer/producer of *Grey's Anatomy*

"*Game On!* is transformative for many reasons, but what I love most about it is: even if you lose, you win. Plus, Az is inspiring and Krista is FUNNY. Have you ever read a health book that really made you laugh? No. You haven't. You're lying if you said yes. But this one will make you laugh."
—Michaela Watkins, actor, *Saturday Night Live*

"The thing about *Game On!* is you can use it to accomplish whatever you want. You want to get in shape? Done. You want to eat right? Done. You want to learn how to prioritize the important things in your life? Done. It's like the perfect mix of your favorite board game, a great workout, and the kick in the ass we all need from time to time."
—Peter Paige, actor, *Queer as Folk*

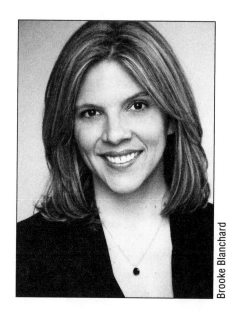

Brooke Blanchard

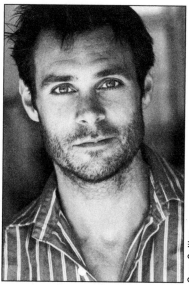

Greg Collins

# About the Authors

KRISTA VERNOFF is the Emmy-nominated head writer and executive producer of television's hit show *Grey's Anatomy*. A playwright and TV writer for the past decade, she holds a BFA from Boston University's College of Fine Arts. She lives in Los Angeles with her husband, Kevin Maynard, and their daughter, Cosette, her proudest accomplishment to date.

AZ FERGUSON is Body-*for*-LIFE's million-dollar champion. After winning the biggest prize money in the history of the health and fitness industry, he moved from his hometown of Sydney, Australia, to his new home in Los Angeles, California, to fulfill a lifelong dream of living in "the land of the free." He has found his true passion in exploring health and fitness as a way of helping people meet their true potential.

# THE
# GAME ON!
## DIET

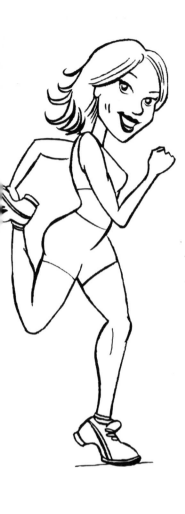

Krista Vernoff

and

Az Ferguson

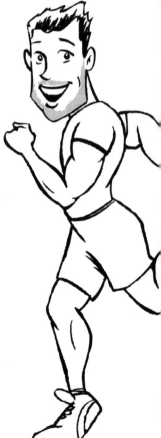

# THE
# GAME
# ON!
# DIET

Kick Your Friend's Butt
While Shrinking Your Own

HARPER

NEW YORK • LONDON • TORONTO • SYDNEY

# HARPER

This book is written as a source of information only. The information contained in this book should by no means be considered a substitute for the advice, decisions, or judgment of the reader's physician or other professional advisor.

All efforts have been made to ensure the accuracy of the information contained in this book as of the date published. The author and the publisher expressly disclaim responsibility for any adverse effects arising from the use or application of the information contained herein.

Illustrations © 2009 Stacy McKee
Art by Stacy McKee and graphic design by Andie Skovron, Bluedog Design
Title page art © Michael Ahern

HarperCollins books may be purchased for educational, business, or sales promotional use. For information please write: Special Markets Department, HarperCollins Publishers, 10 East 53rd Street, New York, NY 10022.

FIRST EDITION

Designed by Joy O'Meara

Library of Congress Cataloging-in-Publication Data is available upon request.

ISBN 978-0-06-171889-2

12 13   OV/RRD   15 14 13 12 11

It is a happy talent to know how to play.

—*Ralph Waldo Emerson*

For Kimberly Skeens, who helped me go from there to here.

And for Kevin and Coco, who make here the happiest place on earth.

—*Krista*


For my mother, Pam Ferguson, my rock,
whose love makes me feel like a giant.

For my father, Michael; one could not ask for a greater mentor.

And for my sister Jasmin, who has always celebrated my life even when I,
being the naughty brother, forgot to celebrate hers.

—*Az*

# Contents

# Contents

# Foreword

**This is not** really a diet book. I hate diets. Everyone I know hates diets. Diets are stupid and hard and not fun, and worse than that, they rarely work. I can only pull my theory on why they don't work from my own experience, which is that they suck and are stupid and not fun. But more than that, if you have any rebellious spirit in you whatsoever, you're gonna rebel against the deprivation of a diet. And whether you rebel at the beginning, the middle, or the end of the diet, the results will be the same: you'll eat like crazy and refuse to move your butt an inch off the couch for weeks. You'll undo any good you may have done, and, if you're like me, you'll end up fatter, flabbier, unhappier, and with lower self-esteem than you had when you started.

Maybe you're not like me; maybe you're like my coauthor, Az, and you thrive on restraint and restriction and deprivation. And if so, yay you, and we can still be friends. (I only hate Az and resent his discipline, like, fourteen percent of the time.) My point is, this book is not going to offer you any fads, any extremes, any swanky new science that says if you eat only protein, or only citrus, or only peanut butter, or only watermelon (all diets I've tried at some point, by the way) you will drop seven sizes in two days. (If that's what you're looking for, we can't help you. Good luck, God bless, return this book now and get your money back. We'll miss you.)

This book isn't even so much about encouraging weight loss as it is about encouraging health and an attitude that will allow you to accomplish healthy weight loss if that's your goal, or toning up if that's your goal, or getting up off your couch for the first time in three years if that's your goal. Truly, I think you're great just the way you are. But if you're not feeling so great, I think the super-fun game you're about to play will help.

I should note here that I am not anything resembling a doctor (though I write some on TV) and neither is Az. Az is really into fitness and we are friends and we played a game together and it made us healthier and now we want to share it with you. Any health advice we offer in this book is coming from copious research and conversations we had with people who are much better educated than we are in the fields of medicine and health (and we have credited those people throughout the book).

Az invented this game to help me lose weight and feel better about myself. Isn't he a good friend? I had a baby a while back (the world's most amazing baby) and while I was pregnant I gained fifty pounds. Fifty. 5-0. 'Cause that's what happens when you're nauseated from the time you wake up until the time you go to sleep and the only thing that staves off the nausea is eating something bready every 15 minutes. And like I mentioned, I got the world's most amazing kid out of it and I don't regret any of it, so there. BUT. Four months after giving birth I was still carrying twenty-four of those extra pounds—which maybe wouldn't have bothered me so much except that when I got pregnant, I was already twenty pounds heavier than I'd ever been.

So, I was bigger than is physically comfortable for me. I had nothing in the closet that fit, which might have been okay if I was still steadily losing weight, but I wasn't. In the prior two months, I had lost only two pounds. I figured at the rate of a quarter pound a week, it would take me, like, forty years to lose that weight. (Math: not my thing.) My maternity clothes were too big, everything else was too small, and the extra weight put me in a size that required me to shop in specialty stores, which was not entirely okay with me.

And so I said to Az one day, "Wanna help me lose some weight, oh fitness-guru friend of mine?" And he said sure, and he came over and taught me about healthy meals, and he taught me a kick-ass interval training thing on the stationary bike, and I was all grateful and motivated, 'cause Az is Australian? And he has that lilting accent? Where everything ends in a question? And it's really quite motivating somehow? But then Az left and I had a script to write and I sat back down with my laptop and my donut and that was pretty much that. (Fine. I have exaggerated slightly. I actually did what he said in a very half-assed way for the next three months and during that time I lost four, maybe five pounds.)

Now, Az is one of those people who, if you set him a task, he will accomplish it or die trying. And I think it got his goat that I asked for his help and then didn't really take his advice. But what's fascinating about Az is that he didn't judge me for not trying hard enough; he judged himself for not having found a way to motivate me. So he sent me an e-mail three months later proposing a game: a dieting game. A kick-ass, competitive, team sport sort of dieting game that we would play with our friends.

Now, I am all sorts of competitive. And if you give me someone to compete against? And a team to answer to? It changes *everything.* The meal plan was the same one Az had given me months before. The exercise plan was the same. But everything was different, 'cause now it wasn't about fitting back into my clothes. It was about kicking someone's ass, and maybe fitting back into my clothes as a bonus. And that made *all the difference in the world.*

I suddenly found that it actually *was* possible to find 20 minutes a day to exercise. And on days when I felt like it wasn't possible, all it took was some nagging from my teammates to motivate me. (Especially 'cause we did a girls' team against a boys' team and we really, really wanted to kick some boy butt. And I should mention here that the game is judged on *points won,* not on *weight lost,* which makes a battle of the sexes not only possible and fair but raucously fun.)

On more than one occasion, I came home from a ten-hour work day, put the baby to bed, ate dinner, and watched TV with my husband, and then, at midnight, realized I hadn't exercised, which meant losing serious points for myself and for my team, which meant that there was no way I was going to bed without exercising first. A working mom—a working *writer*—exercising at midnight? I think this may be previously unheard of in the history of the world.

In the past, when faced with the same situation, motivated only by the notion of burning some extra calories and maybe upping my metabolism a little, no *way* was I getting on the bike at midnight. But motivated by my desire to win a game? By my desire to beat my husband (who was on the opposing team)? By a fear of pissing off my teammates and having to hear about it the next day? I got on the freakin' bike.

Night after night after night, I got on the bike. Meal after meal after meal, I stuck to Az's simple plan (which, by the way, never left me feeling hungry or deprived). And four weeks after the game started I was back in my pre-pregnancy clothes. And two weeks after that, they actually fit. And two weeks later, they were loose. Over that initial nine-week game, I lost more than fifteen pounds.

And the thing is, if you like games, this one is a stupid amount of fun. I *loved* taunting my husband when he would lose points for snacking. I *loved* tallying my points at the end of the day and singing my sister Sydni's loser song to him as he went to sleep. ("Hey! Hey! Hey, hey, hey, hey—loser, loser, loser, you are a loser . . .")

## Krista Vernoff, *40 pounds lost*

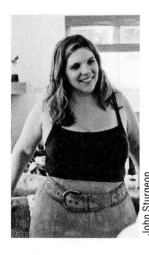
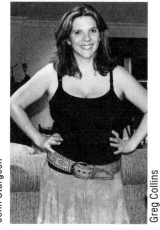
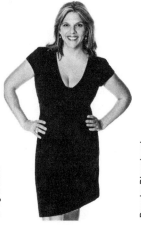

John Sturgeon

Greg Collins

Brooke Blanchard

**Before**              **During**              **After**

But here's the craziest thing: We ended our game on December 20. (The boys' team won, by the way, which I am still not over. Stupid boys.) So after December 20 comes Christmas. And over Christmas we gain weight, right? Except I didn't. What's weirder? I lost three pounds from December 20 to December 31. Without trying. Without even thinking about it. Why? I think it's because, in playing the game, I learned something about food and health and the way my body works. More important, I got in the *habit* of doing things a little differently. So this game is really about helping you change your habits for the better. We just distract you with all the fun. (And by the way, to date, I have lost forty pounds playing the game and I feel better than I have in years.)

All right, that's it. That's my sales pitch. And if you don't want to play, that's cool. No judgment here; I'm sure your life is perfectly happy. But then, I'm kinda laid back about these things. So, for good measure, here's a word from the man himself. Don't forget to read it with that Australian lilt . . .

### • • • A Note from Az • • •

Our health is the key to taking our lives to the next level. It is fundamental to everything we do, to who we are right now and who we can be in the future. Without our health nothing is possible, and so it goes that with only a portion of our health in place, only a portion of what we're capable of is possible.

Optimum health is actually our natural state of being; our bodies naturally gravitate to what they need. Think of a baby in her first year of life. She eats on a regular basis, lots of small meals. She gets most of her meals from fluids, which keep her fully hydrated. She sleeps for large portions of the day to aid her growth and recovery. And when she wakes, she's raring to go!

So what gets in the way of this natural process? We do. We have developed so many belief systems around our health and our bodies and food and exercise and what's right and what's wrong and what's possible. We have so many associations and so much negative conditioning that we end up either extremely confused or just plain resigned to suffer. So we do the bare minimum for our health until we're sick or defeated or both. Just a few years ago, this was true for me. My spine was in such a terrible, painful condition that I'd been advised I needed surgery by three separate doctors. In fact, I had the surgery scheduled. I was terrified by the idea of scalpels slicing into my spine. And then I considered the possibility that my own body, given its fullest opportunity, had the potential to heal itself. I canceled the surgery, and I embarked on building the muscles in my back to better support my spine. Now, that's a bit of an oversimplification of the intense process I took on, but the fact is I didn't have the surgery and just a few months ago, I qualified for the Boston Marathon by completing a marathon in just over three hours. Today, aside from some occasional tightness that I treat with yoga, I am pain free.

I fully committed to my health—to giving it my all—and I changed the course of my life. Now I want to help you change the course of yours.

Playing this game, you'll learn so much about not just your health but also your true self—and you'll have an absolute cracker of a time doing it! No matter what level you're at, Olympic athlete or couch potato, playing the game will take you closer to your optimum health. Oh, and I have to warn you. There is a huge responsibility that goes with the amount of energy and well-being you'll have at the end of this four weeks: You'll no longer have an excuse for not living the life of your dreams! Actually you'll probably have to dream bigger to burn off all the excess energy you'll have!

I hope you play.

I hope you win!

But win or lose, at the end of four weeks, you'll be closer to fulfilling your true potential on this earth—and it doesn't get better than that.

GAME ON PEOPLE, GAME ON!!!

Chapter 1

# HOW TO PLAY THE GAME:
## An Overview

**(Or, I'm Really Too Lazy to Read This Whole Book, Plus, I'm So Out of Shape That Turning Pages Kinda Hurts.)**

You will never win if you never begin.

—*Helen Rowland*

**So, you probably** are gonna have to read a few more chapters to get the hang of this thing. But as with any game, there are some basic rules of play, which we will share with you now. Me, I tend to be that person who, when I get a new board game, I accidentally throw out the rules with the plastic wrapping, and then I just have to make crap up. And so I have learned the hard way that games are usually more fun when played by the *actual* rules than when played by the rules I create in my warped little brain. With that understanding, here are the rules as created in Az's warped little brain. . .

**The object of the game:** To score as many points as possible.

At the end of the game, *the team with the most points wins.*

## Setting Up Your Game

Form two teams or more.

Two players or more per team is ideal.

Teams need not be of equal size (e.g., a team of three can play a team of four).

Each team must designate a Scorekeeper.

## Pick a Prize

Your team and the opposing team must agree on a prize to be awarded to the winning team at the end of the game. The prize can be material (tickets to a show) or service-oriented (driving the carpool for a month, doing the winners' laundry for a month). The prize must be significant (it should hurt a little to lose).

## Choose a Start Date

All team members must agree on a start date. Because each week allows for a day off and a meal off, all holidays can be fully celebrated and impending holidays should not be prohibitive to starting the game.

# How to Play

The game is played for four consecutive weeks.

Each player must use the enclosed score sheet to tally his/her total points per week. Each week, the point tallies must be reported to the team's scorekeeper. The scorekeeping is based on an honor system—*integrity is essential.*

## Keeping Score

A perfect day is worth 100 points. A perfect day includes:

- 30 Meal Points: You earn 6 points per meal for eating five fully sanctioned meals. No snacks between meals.
- 20 Exercise Points: You earn your exercise points by doing some form of exercise for 20 minutes per day.
- 10 Water Points: You earn your water points by drinking three liters of water per day.
- 15 Sleep Points: You earn your sleep points by sleeping for a minimum of seven hours a night.
- 20 Transformation Points: You earn 10 points a day for practicing one healthy new habit and another 10 points a day for eliminating one unhealthy old habit.
- 5 Communication Points: You earn your communication points by being in contact with at least one teammate and at least one opponent each day. (Phone calls, e-mails, and text messages count.)

## Exceptions

Each week, each player gets one meal off in addition to one day off. The meal off and day off may be taken at any time during a given week. They may *not* be saved and carried over into later weeks.

Your day off includes a respite from all rules. This respite may be spread throughout the week (i.e., Monday can be your water day off; Tuesday can be your habits day off; Wednesday can be your sleep day off, etc; or you can take one whole day off from everything).

## Bonus Points

You can also earn a 10-point bonus each week by turning in your scores to your team's scorekeeper by a designated time (e.g., noon on Monday).

In addition, each week, a bonus equaling 20 percent of your points earned for the week is awarded for losing 1 percent of your body weight. (Note: If weight loss is not a goal for you, you must set yourself a fitness goal for which you will win your bonus points and inform your teammates and opponents in advance of beginning the game.)

## Penalties

There is a 10-point Snacking Penalty for snacking between meals.

There is a 20-point Collusion Penalty. If any player suggests to any other player a compromise of integrity, e.g., saying to an opponent, "If I eat a snack and *you* eat a snack, then we both lose points and it all balances out!" the player suggesting the compromise loses 20 points.

There is a 25-point *per portion* Alcohol Penalty. A portion equals any amount of alcohol up to 6 ounces of wine, 12 ounces of beer, or 1.5 ounces of hard liquor. One portion of alcohol may be consumed with the meal off without penalty. Alcohol may be consumed freely on the day off.

If during any week of play a player fails to earn their weight-loss/fitness bonus, that player loses the privilege of alcohol on the day off *for the rest of the game.*

# Winning the Game

At the end of each week, each player turns in their score to the scorekeeper.

A maximum-score week equals seven 100-point days + the 20 percent weight-loss/fitness bonus + the 10-point scorekeeping bonus.

$$700 + 140 = 840 + \text{10-point scorekeeping bonus} = 850$$

A score of 850 points is the (hard to earn!) maximum points for each week.

At the end of each week, the scorekeeper tallies the total points for the team.

The total score for the team is then divided by the number of players on the team.

Example:

Team A has three players. During Week 1, Player 1 earns 750 points. Player 2 earns 850 points. Player 3 earns 780 points.

$750 + 850 + 780 = 2380$

2380 is then divided by 3 for a team score of 793 points.

Team B has 2 players. Player 1 earns 685 points. Player 2 earns 750 points.

$685 + 750 = 1435$

1435 is then divided by 2 for a team score of 717.5.

So at the end of Week 1, Team A is in the lead!

At the end of four weeks, each team's scorekeeper tallies points for the game.

Example:

| Team A | Team B |
|---|---|
| Week 1: 793 points | Week 1: 717.5 points |
| Week 2: 760 points | Week 2: 845 points |
| Week 3: 840 points | Week 3: 810 points |
| Week 4: 800 points | Week 4: 795 points |
| **Total:** 3193 points | **Total:** 3167.5 points |

So at the end of the entire game, Team A has won.

## Tie-Breakers

In the unlikely case of a tie, the game goes to the team with the highest number of 100-point days.

# Results

As a result of the game, your clothes will be looser, your energy will be higher, and you will be losing a minimum of 1 percent of your body weight per week. If any of these things are not true for you after any week of play, please see Chapter 16, Troubleshooting.

Okay, those are the rules. And playing is even easier than it looks. And way more fun. And though very few calories are burned by turning pages, there's a lot of great information in the ensuing chapters. So—after you call all your friends and challenge them to a game—read on. 'Cause then you'll be sure to win. Especially if you, like, withhold a whole bunch of information from your friends. That would be hilarious. You should be all, "No, I swear, you're supposed to eat chocolate cake four times a day!" Hee. Evil. Forget it. Just win fair and square. You can do it. I believe in you.

# Chapter 2

# WHY SHOULD
# I PLAY THE GAME?

**(Or, I Like Myself Just the Way I Am.
Except for the Love Handles. And the Self-Loathing.)**

There are two great days in a person's life—
the day we are born and
the day we discover why.

—*William Barclay*

**My inner feminist** needs to take a moment here to be clear about something: "unhappy" and "fat" do not necessarily always go together even though our culture tries really hard to equate "skinny" with "happy" in the minds of young girls. Two weeks after my dad died, I broke up with my boyfriend of four years. I was the saddest I have ever been in my life. I had some time off, and I went to a yoga retreat for two weeks—mostly because I had promised my dad I would quit smoking and this seemed like a good way to do it. It was four hours of yoga a day, and I lost a bunch of weight and I got a lot of compliments and everyone thought I looked just great, and meanwhile, I was grief-stricken and miserable and pissed that I had quit smoking and that my dad seemed to be staying dead and that I was suddenly single and about to turn thirty. The word "unhappy" doesn't quite do this era justice. But I was thin.

Not long after that, I fell in love with the man who is now my husband. He was training for a triathlon at the time and eating like a person who is training for a triathlon—which is to say, he was eating A LOT of highly caloric foods. Being madly in love, I was happily eating with him, but not training with him. I gained weight and he still thought I was sexy and I loved him more and I was so incredibly happy (despite the fact that my dad seemed to be staying stubbornly dead). So, Young Girls, listen up! There is a reason for the phrase "fat and happy." It's because sometimes a little extra cush is borne of a little extra happy, and sometimes, that's a beautiful thing. So please don't think I'm judging your fat. But if you bought this book, I'm thinking you're at the point of being *unhappy* about the fat because when I was a little fat and very happy, I wasn't buying this kind of book.

So, the title of this chapter poses a question that I can't answer. I really don't know why you should play this game; I only know that you picked this book up off the shelf, which means that you probably know why you should play. I figure the best I can do is tell you why *I* played—and why I continue to play. And the answer to that question goes back way further than my pregnancy and my weight gain in recent years. It's going to involve some over-sharing, by the way. It's also going to involve a little pop quiz for you that goes like this: If you can answer, "Hey, me too!" to even one of my reasons, then this game is definitely for you.

Okay, the over-sharing shall now commence. Buckle your seatbelt and get some popcorn. Wait. This is a diet book. Don't get popcorn.

When I was about four, there was a cereal commercial that asked the question, "Can you pinch an inch?" The commericial made it very clear that the ability to pinch an inch was not a good thing. So I pulled up my shirt and tried it. Oh. Oh no. Panic set in. I could pinch, like, five inches. Now that I think about it, I was probably grabbing my internal organs, but I swear, there were many, many inches of what I thought was unacceptable flab.

I knew that it was unacceptable because not only had the commercial told me so, but my mom had, albeit unintentionally, told me so too. Again, not on purpose. But after a very angry divorce, she had on more than one very angry occasion ranted to her friends about my "fat fuck of a father" and what a pig he was. And then, on far less angry occasions, people told me how much I looked like my dad, how I had "the Vernoff belly." They were saying it lovingly. Many of the people saying it were Vernoffs, after all. But I was no dummy. I could put two and two together. If my dad was a fat fuck and I looked like him . . . I could pinch waaay too many inches.

☑ **Reason #1:** I developed body issues early in life. The issues were unrelated to the actual condition of my body.

**The game takes the focus off of the "issues" and puts the focus on getting healthy, winning points, and having fun.**

*I play because I am determined not to cross the "40" line wearing size 40 jeans and because I would rather have a six-pack than drink one, but in order for that to happen I need some serious motivation, because no matter how many promises I make at 9 a.m., I will have no will power at 9 p.m. unless there is something on the line.*

—Peter, 39

Here's what else: My dad kept the opposite kind of kitchen from my health food vegetarian mom. He shopped—I shit you not—at 7-Eleven. Hot dogs and frozen burritos and Hostess donuts and Slurpees reigned supreme. Kraft Macaroni & Cheese was an impressive cooking feat. And because I got to see my dad only every other weekend, I came to equate the junk food with the good times with my dad and my mom's health food with the ho-hum every day.

My mom cooked delicious soups and kept fresh fruits and veggies around at all times, but junk foods had the lure of forbidden fruit. I remember racing to my friends' cupboards and shoving cookies and candy into my mouth at every opportunity. When I was eight and my sister was ten, we saved up our allowance and went to the grocery store and bought a box of Cookie Crunch and a box of Froot Loops and kept them hidden in the garden shed and would hide out there every day after school, eating it by the handful. (And when our stepdad found the cereal and asked us about it, we said it belonged to the Mormon kids down the street whose parents didn't feed them enough. Hehe. Hee.)

I also remember that for several months before we got caught, my sister and I would *walk across a six-lane highway to get to the gas station on the other side and buy candy.* We were playing a death-defying game of human Frogger for Whoppers and Milk Duds. As a parent? This story is less funny to me than it used to be.

☑ **Reason #2:** I formed very unhealthy food habits very early on in life.

**The game empowered me to begin to replace those habits with happier, healthier habits (and still let me have candy sometimes).**

*I played because I'm a workaholic and I needed desperately to do something different—something that prioritized me and my health for once. I'm not gonna lie—the game takes time and energy and at first I thought I didn't have it to give. But in the end—actually, after only a few days—it was so worth it.*

—Katy, 42

Around puberty, I went on my first diet. And then I went on another diet and then another. All of them failed and/or left me heavier than when I'd started. This is not surprising, because I did not understand what I was doing and I was making up many of the "diets" myself. "I will eat ONLY watermelon because I like it and I heard it's super low-calorie!" "I will eat ONLY grapefruit." (Man, that one wreaked havoc on my skin.) "I will eat ONLY spaghetti. It's fat free!" And eventually: "I will eat nothing and become anorexic like that chick on the track team who's in the hospital!" That lasted seven hours. Thank God, I am not nearly type-A enough for anorexia.

☑ **Reason #3:** I tend to go to extremes—all or nothing.

**The game teaches and rewards balance.**

*I played because I had no clue what I was doing when it came to health and fitness. I knew what I wanted to look like, I just didn't know how to get there. After playing the game I feel confident with food and exercise choices.*

—Kristen, 19

That was high school but things didn't get much better in college. Set free from my mom's healthy kitchen, I gained the Freshman Fifteen and then some. Late night chicken wings in the dorm were my undoing. And every time I got on the scale, I'd be all, "But I only drink DIET Coke!" Then after my junior year, I tried the "all booze and cigarettes" diet. That one was fun, and I lost a bunch of weight, until I landed in the hospital with a kidney infection that went into my bloodstream and almost killed me. Sepsis! Not fun! I do not recommend it!

☑ **Reason #4:** I have a very sneaky mind. I can justify almost any behavior and convince myself it has health benefits.

The game teaches and reinforces the body basics you need to make healthy, life-sustaining, weight-dropping, self-esteem-building choices.

*I played because I have been thin my whole life until this past year when I gained so much weight that I laughed every time I looked in the mirror . . . I truly did not recognize myself! None of my clothes fit. I tried many diets and only got fatter. The game looked like a lifestyle change not just a fad diet and I was willing to try anything. I lost ten pounds and it has stayed off. In fact I have stayed with the diet and I have lost an additional five pounds. The best thing that came from the game is the fact that my blood pressure has continually gone down. I have cut my medication in half and it is still going down. I look forward to even-tually doing away with the medication altogether. The game wasn't just the answer to my weight problem but it has turned out to be the answer to my health as well. Thanks!*

*—Chris, 54*

Now let's talk about numbers for a minute. REAL numbers.

I am 5'7" with hefty Ukrainian bones. When I graduated high school, I was about a size 8 at 150 pounds. Healthy. My freshman year of college, I topped out at 166. The summer after my junior year, I waited tables on a three-story harbor cruise ship, burned a ton of calories going up and down the stairs (and smoked a lot instead of eating), and got down to 140 pounds (which is about a size 6 and as thin as I should ever be). When I graduated from college, I was in the range of 150 again. Waiting tables in New York and eating pasta for free every night, I put on a few pounds. Living in Portland after that, I naturally struck a pretty healthy balance be-tween eating and exercise and my weight held steady at about 155.

In 1998, at about 155 pounds and the age of twenty-seven, I moved to L.A. to be a writer. And by the time I got pregnant at the age of thirty-four, I weighed *185 pounds* (and this was after spending a week at a juice spa to "cleanse" in preparation for pregnancy). Why the huge jump? Because of the physical complacency of a writer's life. Most days, I sit in a room talk-ing for ten hours, which burns way fewer calories than I wish it did. Also, lifting your arm to hoist cookies into your mouth? Doesn't burn so many calories either, and that was my main other activity in the writer's room. When I'm not in the writer's room, I'm in an easy chair in my office with a computer on my lap. Many days, if I'm veeeeery quiet, I can hear the cellulite growing.

☑ **Reason #5:** I had become complacent and complacency had led to laziness. I was unable to even imagine a world in which exercise was a daily possibility.

The game motivates you to come up with exercise time every day and teaches you how to maximize the time you have.

*I played because after a few years being married and lazy I had become a fat bastard. When I jumped in the pool, kids ducked for cover.*
                                                              —Kevin, 41

Of course, by the time I got pregnant I didn't even know how much I weighed, because I had not stepped on a scale *in years*. The first time I went to the obstetrician and she wanted to weigh me, I faced away from the scale. I thought that if I avoided the number, I could avoid the self-esteem crash. (In the end I found that all I was doing by avoiding the number was perpetuating the denial that allowed me to get that big to begin with.)

So how do I know now what I weighed then? Around week 35 of pregnancy my doctor accidentally left the scale in place instead of zeroing it out before I could see it. And so I was lying on the table, and I looked over and saw that the big weight was on 200. If *that* wasn't enough to make a person cry and pretend she's having an allergy attack, the little weight was at 28. 228. TWO HUNDRED AND TWENTY-EIGHT POUNDS. I stopped breathing. How on earth could I weigh 228?? The last time I had actually checked I was around 160! Still, by the end of my pregnancy I weighed 235 pounds. Twenty-five of those pounds fell off that first week after giving birth. The rest lingered. The "before" picture you've seen in this book is me at around 210 pounds. I look at it and I don't recognize myself. (And if you're thinking, "Holy crap! I can't believe she put that picture in this book for all her ex-boyfriends and the world to see! That's, like, the bravest, craziest thing I've ever seen!" You are correct. Brave and fucking CRAZY.)

☑ **Reason #6:** I had spent years lying to myself about my actual weight.

The game asks you to dust off the scale and give yourself all the information. Having all the information is empowering.

*I play because I am a vain gay man. No, seriously, I play because in my twenties, my body played cruel tricks on me and allowed me to eat whatever donut, fat burger, or fried piece of goodness that my heart desired. But as I entered my thirties and my habits remained the same, I suddenly realized that every extra calorie made an appearance around my once-tiny little waist. So I had to train my body to actually work for me instead of against me. It was extremely tough at first, but let me tell you, I am loving my new thirty-year-old healthy body.*

—Brad, 32

What's funny is, a lot of years of therapy and the incredibly life-changing event of having a baby healed a lot of what was broken for that "fat fuck" of a four-year-old. At 210 pounds, I was speaking to myself far more kindly than I ever did at 150. It became abundantly clear to me that self-esteem has veeeery little to do with the number on the scale or the size of the clothes. It is, as they say, "an inside job." At 210 pounds, I was happier—*truly happier*—than I had ever been. I had a baby. An amazing, hilarious, giggly, farty, burpy bundle of happy, healthy baby. And a wonderful husband and a job I loved (and a lovely eleven-week maternity leave).

I was exquisitely blessed.

I was also obese.

When I asked Az for help to lose the weight, it was primarily because I did not feel well *physically*. My knees hurt and my back hurt and my energy was low and I felt older than my years despite all that happiness. So when Az taught me the five-meal-a-day plan and the interval training exercises you're about to see outlined in this book, I really thought, *hell, yes, I'm gonna take this on!*

And then I didn't. Or I did, but *really* half-heartedly. (Quarterheartedly?) So this time, the diet wasn't failing because of a shame cycle, or lack of information. It was failing because my life was way more interesting than the diet. It was failing because it bored me and I would way rather gaze at my baby than get on a bike.

And the game changed all of that. The game was fun. The game was fierce. The game gave me permission to diet openly, aggressively, in-your-face-ively, which is my new favorite word that I just made up. Whereas before I had been mortified by the number on the scale, I was now shouting at anyone who'd listen. *"Hey! Guess what?? I weighed 199 last week and now I'm only 195!! I'm only 195 and next week I'M GONNA WEIGH LESS!"* The whole thing was fun. And I lost a whole lot of weight and that was *really* fun.

☑ **Reason #7:** I find dieting boring.

The game is fun!

*I play because left to my own devices I am a lazy, cookie-eating, chip-craving madman with a bicycle tire around my midsection.*

—M.P., 39

So these are my stories. (Okay, fine, I have more stories, but I gotta save some for the rest of the book.) But these are my reasons for playing.

What are yours?

Food, weight, weight loss . . . these are not simple subjects in our culture.

I have met very few people who don't have painful weight stories or crazy diet stories or screwed up parents and mean ex-boyfriends that led to painful weight stories and crazy diet stories.

So tell your stories.

Tell your secrets.

Tell them to your spouses and tell them to your friends.

And if you're not ready to do that, then start by telling them to yourself.

The game you are about to play is pulling dieting out of the closet. It's making it a group sport. It is acknowledging that we are all a little fucked in the head—so why not just talk about it?

Tell your story. Because it's the answer to why you should play this game.

## GET A PEN!

Right now, write down some of your own reasons for wanting to play this game. Be brutally honest. This is only for you.

-------------------------------------------------------

-------------------------------------------------------

-------------------------------------------------------

-------------------------------------------------------

-------------------------------------------------------

-------------------------------------------------------

-------------------------------------------------------

-------------------------------------------------------

-------------------------------------------------------

-------------------------------------------------------

-------------------------------------------------------

-------------------------------------------------------

-------------------------------------------------------

-------------------------------------------------------

-------------------------------------------------------

-------------------------------------------------------

-------------------------------------------------------

-------------------------------------------------------

-------------------------------------------------------

-------------------------------------------------------

# Chapter 3

# TEAMING UP

## (Or, Why Should I Give a Crap What Anyone Else Does?)

The strength of the team
is each individual member . . .
the strength of each member is the team.

—*Phil Jackson*

**In grade school** and in middle school and in high school, I was the kid chosen last whenever there was any kind of team game. I know we all like to joke about how we were the kid chosen last—but really, most of you weren't dead last. You were maybe fifth to last, or third to last, and it just felt like you were last because you wanted to be first. I was *actually last*. I was chosen after the kids with various physical and mental disabilities. *Every time.*

It's not just that I was horribly unpopular; it's that I was teeeeeerrible at sports. I had an uncommon combination of a total lack of skill and a total lack of interest. I was generally living inside my head, writing stories, planning my Oscar acceptance speech, or imagining what I might say to the cute boy on second base if he ever noticed I was alive. If, God forbid, the ball came my way, I was lucky if I noticed in time to duck.

One of my most vivid childhood memories is from the first grade when I was, as usual, chosen last for the softball game. I went up to bat with my usual combination of disinterest and terror—and I actually *hit the ball* and *ran to first base*. It was my own private miracle. It was like the bat moved all by itself and then a swift wind came and pushed me to the base. Then, in an even more stunning turn of events, I actually made it, one hitter at a time, one base at a time, all the way back to home plate and scored! *I was actually cheered on by my team!* I went home and told my mom I had hit a home run, because that is what I believed I had done. (I actually didn't understand the difference between making it home and hitting a home run till, like, last year.) I was very, very proud. If you're expecting that where this story goes is that I became strung out on the feeling and got better at team sports, you are wrong. I just figured a "home run" was all anyone could ever expect of me, and that was the last effort I put into any kind of team sport, ever.

> *I loved the game because there aren't a lot of competitions that I stand a good chance of actually winning. With the game, it was just mind over matter. Plus wanting to kick some serious ass.*
>
> —Emily, 27

But games? Games are another thing entirely. I am a highly competitive game-player. Like, during friendly games of Celebrity and Taboo I've been known to become so intense and scream so loudly, I've made people cry. I was reading about game theory when I started writing this book and I read that there are fundamentally two different types of game-players: there are social players, who really don't care if they win or lose and are just happy to have fun playing, and then there's me.

I do not like to lose.

Whether this comes from a childhood of being chosen last or from the fact that I am a Scorpio with Sagittarius rising, I don't know. I just know that if you play on my team, you'd better not play lightly. I'm not saying you shouldn't have fun. Have all the fun you want, just don't fuck me up while you do. Because—did I mention? I LIKE TO WIN.

Az noticed this. Which is why he invented this game for me. I may have mentioned this already, but I think it bears repeating that Az gave me the food and exercise plan in July, and from July to October, I lost five pounds. And then we started playing the game. And from October to December, I lost fifteen pounds. Same food plan. Same exercise plan. The only difference was that I was doing it for points. And I was doing it for my team. And I was doing it against someone else's team. Which prompted me to actually DO IT. The team aspect made a huge difference to me. I was motivated by winning, sure, but I was also motivated by the desire to support/please/not piss off my team. And as it turns out, there are actual studies to back this up . . .

A weight-loss study published in 2001 indicates that *groups can achieve better results than one-on-one interventions*. Even when the study participants *preferred* individual treatment, they saw better results in group settings, losing 11 percent of their weight compared with 9 percent for individuals.

In another study, dieters who attended weekly support-group sessions had lower cortisol levels than dieters who dieted alone. How crazy is that? That by meeting with other dieters once a week, people were literally, physically, biologically less stressed out??

> *My team won! We beat six other teams in an all-out brawl. I didn't really know these women when I started—one was the niece of my best friend, one was a casual acquaintance—but by the end, they felt like sisters. Every time we talked I was amazed by how much we had in common despite a twenty-year age spread between us. We shared recipes, we shared frustrations, and occasionally we shared a meal off. We supported each other and as a result, we not only won the game, but for the first time in all of our lives, we felt like we were in charge of our diets and our bodies and our health. And beating all those guys was AWESOME.*
>
> —Jesse, 37

One more thing about playing with and against teams: It's FUN. If you're playing all out, your e-mail box will be loaded every morning with messages like, "EAT A CUPCAKE! EAT ONE! YOU KNOW YOU WANT ONE!" And you'll be all, "Screw him. I'm not eating a cupcake! I will instead spend my morning composing pithy poems about my opponents!"

Some actual e-mails during our months of gaming . . .

*Note: During this particular game, we had color-coded our teams, as you will see . . .*

knock, knock,
who's there?

banana.

banana who?

knock, knock,

who's there?

banana.

banana who?

knock, knock,

who's there?

orange.

orange who?

ORANGE IS GONNA KICK YOUR ASS, THAT'S WHO

Love, Anselm

Dear Anselm,

Orange is the color of baby poo after they eat carrots. Red is the color of victory.

Krista

What color am I? Is "winning team" a color? 'Cause it looks great on me.

Doug

I think this Anselm dude has been drinking . . .

I would say "White will Win" but it sounds horribly racist.

Michael

I must admit, I *was* drunk last night.

Drunk with the power that comes from a perfect points day. And already meeting my weight goal for the week.

Orange don't take no mess.

Anselm

So what have we learned from the above? Well, for one thing, we've learned that everyone is more clever in their trash talk than I. "The color of baby poo after they eat carrots?" Seriously? That's the best I could do?? That's just lying down on the job, is what that is.

Also, we have learned that taunting is encouraged. Taunting is encouraged because the game is meant to be fun and taunting is fun and funny and, strangely, motivating.

BUT the game is also meant to create a support system for your health goals. So ONLY play with people you know will have your best interests at heart. ONLY play with people you like and respect and trust to be supportive. Funny is one thing. Unkind is wholly another. You want everyone in your game, teammates and opponents, to be willing to drop all sense of competition if you are needing a few kind words of support. It's like in sports, when a player goes down on the field, the players on both teams stop playing and help him up. It's good sportsmanship, and it must be applied to this game as well. So, here's another series of actual e-mails from that very same game:

Hey everyone! I just wanted to tell you that I've lost 4 pounds this week, and the biggest joy about that was going running yesterday 4 pounds lighter! HOLY CRAP!!! It's so much easier to run with that weight gone!! It's motivation for sure to keep going.

Thank you all for your support (even though it looks somewhat nastier than any kind of support I've ever had).

Ok. Gotta go run 10 MILES and kick all your asses!!!

Kate

Kate—proud of you!

Michael

Kate—rock on. You will still lose, of course, but please lose knowing you have all my respect.

**O**utstanding

**R**esults

**A**re

**N**ever

**G**ained

**E**asily

ORANGE ORANGE ORANGE!!!!

Anselm

So let's talk now about how you find people to play with you. If your plan is to go get the three fattest people you can find and challenge them to a game, heh, I like your thinking. It's never fun to acknowledge your back fat to people who are skinnier than you. But here's what I know: My skinny friends have their share of issues just like the rest of us. They look at their gorgeous bodies and they don't feel good, just like the rest of us. They feel defeated by what to me is an invisible layer of flab around their belly, just like the rest of us feel defeated by our larger rolls of flab. Our bodies may look different but the way we feel about our bodies is remarkably similar no matter what our size.

How do I know this? For starters, I know it because I've been a lot of different weights in my life. When I look at pictures of myself in high school, I am amazed and saddened to remember how much I hated my body and how fat I thought I was. I would kill for that body now. I had a great rack and fantastic legs—and yeah, I had a curvy belly because I inherited my curvy belly from both sides of my family and *there is no weight at which I don't have it*. I wish so much that I had understood that in my teens and twenties. My beautiful assistant, Star, is twenty-two and just gorgeous and I plead with her daily to appreciate what she has, and, of course, she can't, because we are all so fucked in the head.

Contemporary society has fucked us. The starlets on the magazine covers have fucked us. Kate Moss almost singlehandedly fucked my entire generation. "*Heroine chic?*" Jesus Christ, we are fucked in the heads. And I am ranting . . . And I can't remember what I was talking about . . . Hang on . . . Oh, right. Teaming up. Okay, I will now make an attempt to gracefully bring this topic full circle . . .

Being built like me, it's easy to want to dismiss the body woes of my skinnier friends and assume that they don't need and shouldn't want to play this game. But when I do that, I'm missing the point, which is that almost all of us struggle with our bodies, no matter what our size. And it's important to remember that the game is not only about getting fit, it's also about getting healthy. And one of the many things I love about it is that it evens the playing field. Someone built like me can play against someone built like Az and sometimes I win, and sometimes he wins, and we always both win because we are always healthier and feel better when the game is over than when it started.

So, now that we are agreed that almost everyone you know could benefit from playing, I will say that I think the best place to start looking for players is at home, because if you can get a household game going, you're more likely to eliminate the unhealthy foods from your fridge. So maybe start by challenging your husband or wife or girlfriend or boyfriend or sister or brother or parent to a game. (Depending on the dynamics in your relationship, you can either play on the same team or play against each other. You decide.) Once you've got one person on board, you can both ask other family members, as well as your neighbors, your friends, your friends' spouses, your coworkers, the moms and dads in your carpool, your gym buddy, your children's friends' parents, or just about anyone else you can think of.

## Step Up Your Game!

Get an office game going!

Even those of us who've committed to a healthier lifestyle and filled our fridge with fruits and veggies tend to slack off at the office. Someone brings a box of donuts, someone has a birthday cake, someone makes a coffee run and the next thing you know you're ordering Fudgeaccinos and licking frosting off your fingers. So challenge your office mates to a game. Whether you get everyone playing and form two huge teams, or just get three or four coworkers on board, you'll be amazed how much easier it becomes to resist temptation!

**Bonus idea:** Make the prize at the end a month of freedom from the most loathed job in the office. For example, the winners don't have to refill the paper in the copier, or run for the boss' coffee, or drive the carpool for a month. Bought prizes are great, but the kind you can't buy tend to be even more motivating!

*I recently interviewed for a new financial advisor for my company. The last guy that came in was perfect and I offered him the position starting Wednesday. He graciously accepted with one condition. He wanted to start on Monday. He said "One of your coworkers told me about "Game On" while I was waiting for the interview and I didn't want to miss out on the next round." I guess he's one more person whose butt I'm going to have to kick! I'm 15 pounds down and counting!*

—Moj, 30

Word to the wise: Be very careful when you invite people to play that they don't think you're calling them fat. Many of the people I've played this game with do not qualify as fat under *anyone's* definition. Az, for example, has no freaking body fat, but we're two weeks into a new game as I write this. Why? Because he's training for the Boston Marathon. He uses the game as added motivation to run all those miles every day. Believe it or not, we're also using the game to write this book! Az's healthy habit (see Chapter 12) is to work on this book for a minimum of three hours every day. He loses points if he doesn't do it, so he does it. This is not just a diet game, it's a better-life game, a goal-meeting game, a health-improving game—it's whatever kind of game you need it to be. So don't be shy, ask your friends and family to play. (But when you do, show them Az's picture and say, "this guy's playing," just for good measure.)

Okay, so now that you know how to build a team, how the hell are you supposed to work with them? Well, lucky for you I've been playing this game for . . . um . . . ever. And I have gleaned some experience in how best to make this whole thing work. So without further ado, here are my top ten tips for making the most out of working with your team!

## Teamwork Tips

1. Meet with all your players (teammates and opponents) every weekend for a weigh-in/discourse/day off meal. The meetings keep everyone involved, and the weigh-in keeps everyone honest! Even if you don't want a group weigh-in, have the meeting. It gives

everyone a chance to ask questions and to share strategies, recipes, successes, and challenges. It's invaluable.

2. You can earn your communication points by e-mail or text message, but try actually getting on the phone with a teammate once a day. It's great to actually talk it out—to celebrate your successes and vent your frustrations in a more personal way than typing allows.

3. Have a night out or a meal off with your team. Again, the more cohesive you are as a team, the more responsible you will feel for your scores (and the more driven to kick the opposing team's collective ass!).

4. If you're a wiz in the kitchen, share recipes with your team. (And if you want some really good karma, share them with your opponents as well.)

5. Meet a teammate at the gym or park each day (or even one day a week) for a shared workout. It's always a great way to keep each other accountable and motivated. Better yet, meet an opponent and race them on the treadmill!

6. When you are considering losing snacking points—say, you're overcome with an urge for one of the fresh donuts someone just brought to work—call a teammate! Tell them you're desperate for a donut! It will do three things. First, it'll create a pause, which may be enough to give the craving time to subside. Second, it'll give you an opportunity to talk about whatever it is that's driving you toward that donut. Sure, it could just be a physical craving, but more often, it's a mood or a feeling you're looking to avoid. Talking it out will help. Third, it'll give your teammate a chance to talk you through all the reasons you don't need the donut and shouldn't waste the points (and this may help him or her as much as he or she's helping you).

7. Get together with a teammate each Sunday night and do your cooking for the week. It makes the cooking a social event and that way it doesn't feel like a chore.

8. Write a motivational e-mail to your whole team once a day.

9. Write a funny, smack-talking e-mail to your opponents once a day and cc your whole team. There is nothing to keep everyone going like funny, healthy competitive ranting.

10. Share your successes with your team each day. If you have a perfect or near-perfect day, write or call and brag about it! And even more important, if you have a slip and lose points, write your whole team on the day it happened and explain what happened and why and how. It keeps you accountable and you will be far less likely to do the same thing tomorrow!

### • • • A Tip from Az • • •

Teamwork was the most challenging aspect of this game for me by far. (And yes, contrary to what Krista would have you believe, even I find aspects of this game challenging!) I come from Australia, which means I come from the school that says, "I'll look after my side of things and you guys look after yours." But what I've learned playing this game is, that attitude doesn't work. You absolutely must invest in how each member of your team is doing if you want to win. (And I'm starting to realize this rule applies to life and friendship and love as well as this game!) Check in with your teammates each day. Let them know how you're doing, but more important, ask how they're doing and ask if there's anything you can do today to help them step up their game. Even if you're busy as hell, send a text message of support. It'll make your mate feel good, it'll make you feel great, and it'll help your team make its way to victory!

## Frequently Asked Questions

Q: Is there an ideal number of players for a team?

A: We have found that teams of two, three, or four players are great. When the teams get bigger than that, individual players start to feel less responsibility for their personal scores. (Like, you start to think, "Eh, Kevin and Jody always get great scores, so I can slack off a little and not bring the team down too much.") That said, big games can be very fun and provide a lot of support and community. So, truly, anything goes!

Q: Can I play as a team of one against a team of more than one?

A: Yes, you can, but it's not ideal. The group support is a big part of what makes this game effective and fun.

Q: I think my brother should play because I'm worried about his weight, but I don't really want to play with him, because I don't trust him to be honest and sometimes he says really mean things to me. Should I play with him anyway?

A: Worry about your own health first, then his. Play with people you not only like but also love and respect. As you start to feel and look better, your brother may notice and ask what you've been doing, at which point you can tell him about the game and let him play with his own friends. Do NOT play with him if you don't trust him to be fair and kind. It will only piss you off and sabotage your game (which means sabotage your health).

Q: I have such a long history of failing on diets. I want to play but I am really worried about disappointing my team.

A: Here's the deal: Even if you don't score 100 percent you will be healthier for having played. So there are two things I suggest. First, remember the two types of players? There are people who thrive on winning and there are people who just enjoy playing. Find some of the latter and team up with them. And second, tell your teammates about your fear and then talk to them about WHY you have failed at diets in the past. Was it the late night hours that undid you? Maybe you can make a nightly phone appointment with a teammate and talk through those late night cravings. Was it a loathing of all things exercise-related that undid you? Maybe one of your teammates can become your workout buddy and meet you for a nightly run/walk around your neighborhood. Are you an emotional eater and in the past, bad days and sad feelings led to eating binges? Tell your teammates and ask if you can call them when you feel like eating.

Studies have shown that the act of simply pausing and/or talking when an emotional eating urge hits can abate the urge. This game provides you with a vehicle and a community to work through the issues that have undone you in the past. So play the game and use your team and then revel in the results! Go you! Go go go you!!

Q:   I have read this whole chapter and I hear what you're saying but I know myself and I hate team games. Can't I pleeeeease just play someone one on one? Or better yet, can I play all by myself?

A:   Yeah, you totally can. Read the next chapter; it tells you how.

• • • • • • • • • • • • • • • • • • • • • • • • • • • • • • • • • • • • • • • • •
## Play by the Rules
• • • • • • • • • • • • • • • • • • • • • • • • • • • • • • • • • • • • • • • • •

- Form a team of two players or more and challenge a team of two players or more.
- Your team scores are averaged, so you do not need an even number of players and you can play with and against people who are at different fitness levels than you.
- Your team players are meant to be a source of support, so choose wisely.
- People who have group support tend to lose more weight than those who don't.
- Playful taunting is encouraged. But support of all players is essential.
- Only play with people you know will have your best interests at heart.
- When asking people to participate, remember that the game is not only about getting fit, it's about getting *healthy*.
- When you are looking for game-players, start with the people closest to you at home, or in your various communities.
- You do not have to play with or on a team (but before you make that choice, read the next chapter).

## Richard Maher, *lost 30 pounds*

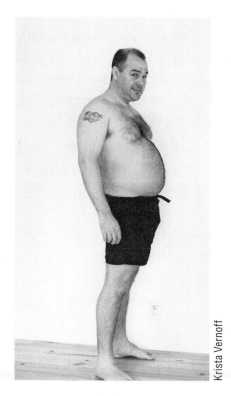
Krista Vernoff

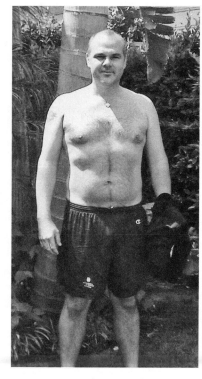
Erin Clendenin

I played the game because I needed to change the way I was doing things. I had a rough five years with the loss of a loved one and a serious neck injury. I put on sixty pounds in those years and could not get them off no matter what I tried. Having always been active in life, the fact that I could not take the weight off reinforced my damaged mental state.

I loved the game because in three months I lost over thirty pounds by EATING MORE THAN I NORMALLY EAT. With this game (a term which seriously underplays what it really is), I know I can get back to my healthy weight without starving myself.

Thank you so much Krista and Az!

Richard, 40

# GET A PEN!

Think about all of the people you know. Then, on the following lines, list ten people off the top of your head who you think might like to play. Then list your top three choices for teammates and why you'd like to play with them and your top three choices for opponents and why you'd like to play against them. E.g.: "I'd like to play with Sally 'cause she's always so supportive," and "I'd like to play against Ralph because I know he will bring the funny trash talk."

_____

_____

_____

_____

_____

_____

_____

_____

_____

_____

_____

_____

_____

_____

_____

_____

_____

_____

_____

_____

_____

_____

# Chapter 4

# PLAYING BY YOURSELF

## (Which Differs Slightly from Playing with Yourself)

And remember,
no matter where you go,
there you are.
—*Confucius*

> **The Rule:** If you don't want to play with a team, find an opponent, agree on a prize, and play. The rules are the same.

**I'm not gonna** lie to you. I was aaaaaalllll prepared to write this chapter as a guilt trip. Like, okay fine, if you *really* can't find a way to be a team player then I *suppose* you can play one on one, but you're kind of a loser if you do. But then, in preparing to write the chapter, I figured we should actually *try* the game one on one. So Az and I played each other, and guess what happened? I got a perfect score three weeks in a row *for the first time ever*.

Then, in week four, I had a psychological collapse surrounding a desperate craving for high-fructose corn sweetener and I lost. I still can't quite talk about it.

Remember the thing about how there are two kinds of players? There are the kind who play to win and the kind who play for the fun of it. If you are the kind who likes to win, and you can find another player who likes to win as much as you do, then playing one on one can be a really fun thing.

> *I took on my wife, who is very type-A and very competitive. She organized the refrigerator for herself—put all her little meals in little Tupperwares—but did not make any for me. After that I decided we should probably play on the same team.*
>
> —Greg, 54

Playing one on one is strangely more intense and more competitive than playing with a team 'cause you have no one to blame but yourself if you fall down. You're Tiger Woods or you're Some Really Famous Tennis Player whose name I don't know 'cause I don't watch tennis. It's just you and the ball and the opponent, and oh, my GOD I'm bad at writing sports metaphors. My husband is going to read this chapter and laaaaaugh. Whatever. 'Cause he is not so good at the one-on-one game.

Not too long ago, I watched him and our friend Adam shake hands at a party. They were both feeling a little fat and wanting a game but not wanting to organize one, so they figured they'd go mano a mano.

They were all pumped up.

They said they were starting Monday.

They bet an expensive dinner.

And that is the last time either of them ever discussed it.

I think they might have been drunk. But, more important, they both played football in high school and college—they are both team sport guys.

A month later, we organized a team game and put them on opposing teams and they both played all out and lost a bunch of weight.

So the trick here is to figure out whether a team will motivate you more than *you* will motivate you. I can say this—the fact that it was a team game inspired and drove me in the beginning. I KNOW I wouldn't have played if Az had initially challenged me to a one-on-one game. But once I fell in love with the game, knew how good it made me feel, knew that it consistently helps me lose weight, I was happy to play one-on-one—I even played better.

## • • • A Tip from Az • • •

Consider playing on a team but taking on a side bet with another player. It can be a player from your own team or the opposing team. Say, "Hey, mate, I bet I get a higher score than you this week. If I do, I win _____, but if you do, you win _____." And bet something BIG. And then, if you tie, push the bet another week and then another. This way, you have team motivation and one-on-one motivation. A perfect combination for a perfect game.

Either way, playing with a team or playing one on one, the rules don't change. But there is one real trick to playing one on one—and that is that you have to act as both competitor and support system for your opponent! You have to trash-talk him one minute and then call to offer support the next. Az and I are like siblings at this point, so this works for us, but choose your opponent carefully if you decide to play one on one because you will need their support!

**But what about playing all by yourself**? Can you just put up a prize, play the game on your own, and promise yourself you'll reward yourself at the end if you reach a certain score?

No.

Fine. Yes.

You can totally do that.

But please do it only AFTER you've played the game the way it's meant to be played at least once. Because the most successful diet and exercise plans ever studied are those that have a group support element.

And also ask yourself just one question: *How well has going it alone worked for me until now?*

There are people who are simply loners and they like it that way. And then there are those who are lonely. I have no studies to back this up, but I have a theory that Loneliness + Time = Extra Fat. So why not reach out? Take a leap. Form a community or just the very beginnings of one. I can tell you that playing by myself doesn't work for me because I absolutely require the competition as motivation, which means a competitor is required. But I do have friends who, after playing a team game, have had "tune up" weeks when they play on their own, challenging themselves to accomplish a certain score, and that has worked for them to lose a few pounds here and there. I'm cool with that.

*A few weeks after playing the game I noticed that I was slacking off a bit. I'd put on a few pounds again and the flab around my stomach was coming back. So I decided to play a mini-game against myself. I drew up the same points system and set myself goals. If I met my targets by the end of the week, I bought two presents: one for myself, and one*

*for my sister. If I didn't meet my targets, she's the only one who'd get*
*a present, and I would have to try again next week. Talk about sibling*
*rivalry being a motivator!*

—Josh, 24

But the idea of your *never* experiencing the game as it's meant to be played—the game as competition and community—makes me sad. 'Cause I feel like you're missing out on something big. And here's the last thing I'll say on this: Az and I have noticed over and over again that the way people play this game tends to reflect the way they live their lives.

Az is an intense, driven perfectionist with the occasional impulse for self-sabotage and his scores tend to reflect that. (Two perfect weeks and then a random series of penalties where he snacks on something like a few grapes and loses a bunch of points for no good reason.)

I tend to be disorganized and chaotic and my scores tend to reflect that. (A perfect day, a semi-crappy day, two perfect days, a crappy day . . .)

Another friend of ours has huge trouble with follow-through in his life—and indeed, he played the game for three weeks and then dropped out for no good reason.

How we play the game reflects how we live our lives.

So if your instinct is to play all alone, thereby missing out on key elements of the game, it makes me wonder what else you're missing out on in your life.

Maybe this is a notion worth considering.

Maybe not.

Who the hell am I, anyway? I'm a TV writer with nothing even resembling a medical degree. So your psychoanalysis for the day will now officially come to a close.

## Frequently Asked Questions

Q:  I like to compete with my husband, but in the past when we've had weight loss contests, he always wins. I think men just lose weight faster. Am I right?

A:   Yes, men do tend to lose weight faster and there are a lot of stud-
      ies currently underway to determine exactly why. Part of it is men
      have more muscle, which helps them burn fat faster. Part of it
      is that women have more estrogen, which helps the body retain
      weight in preparation for pregnancy. But the only really important
      thing here is that YOUR HUSBAND WON'T WIN THIS GAME
      BY LOSING WEIGHT FASTER THAN YOU!!!! It's my favorite
      thing about the game—it isn't won on pounds lost, it's won on
      points earned. Yes, you do have to lose a minimal amount of
      weight each week to earn your bonus points, but if your hubby
      drops ten pounds of water weight week one and you lose more like
      two or three, he doesn't have a leg up on you. It's why I can com-
      pete against Az and occasionally beat him. So go you! Kick that fat
      bastard's ass or die trying! Go go go!

Q:   If I start playing one on one, and then someone wants to join mid-
      game, should I let them?
A:   I see no good reason why not. The more the merrier.

• • • • • • • • • • • • • • • • • • • • • • • • • • • • • • • • • • • • • • • •
## Play by the Rules
• • • • • • • • • • • • • • • • • • • • • • • • • • • • • • • • • • • • • • •

- You can play one on one. Rules stay the same.
- If you are competitive and like to win, playing one on one may be
  more motivating for you.
- Ask yourself if having a team will motivate you or not. If you're not
  sure, try playing with a team first.
- The game is designed to be played with others because of the support a community will give you as you transform your badass self.

# GET A PEN!

Write down the reasons you want to play one on one. Then weigh those against the benefits of playing with a team that I described in the last chapter. Let it be a little pros-and-cons list. If you still think you want to play one on one, then write down the names of a few close friends who might make good one-on-one competitors.

---------------------------------------------------------------

---------------------------------------------------------------

---------------------------------------------------------------

---------------------------------------------------------------

---------------------------------------------------------------

---------------------------------------------------------------

---------------------------------------------------------------

---------------------------------------------------------------

---------------------------------------------------------------

---------------------------------------------------------------

---------------------------------------------------------------

---------------------------------------------------------------

---------------------------------------------------------------

---------------------------------------------------------------

---------------------------------------------------------------

---------------------------------------------------------------

---------------------------------------------------------------

---------------------------------------------------------------

---------------------------------------------------------------

---------------------------------------------------------------

---------------------------------------------------------------

---------------------------------------------------------------

Chapter 5

# PICKING A PRIZE

### (Or, Okay, I'm Skinny, Whatever, but WHAT DO I WIN???)

How you play the game is for college ball.
When you're playing for money,
winning is the only thing that matters.

—*Leo Durocher*

When we were kids, my very athletic sister's room was FILLED with blue ribbons and my room was filled with "Most kids as slow as you would not even show up so good for you for trying!" placards. The first trophy I ever won in my life was the Writers Guild Award for *Grey's Anatomy*. Looking at it, I was overcome with the urge to call my sister and go, "Nah nah nah nah nah!" which makes no sense, because my sister is super supportive and not even a writer. But let's face it: Bragging rights are the real prize in any victory. When the Celtics won the NBA Finals, my husband did not go around saying, "Did you see the size of that trophy???" He went around saying, "Celtics, baby! CEEEELLTIIIIICS!!!" to all of his friends who are Lakers fans.

Tonight, I am going to dinner at a very nice Japanese restaurant of my choosing because my team won the last game I played. (Yes, I have been playing the game on and off for many months now. No, it has not bored me yet. Yes, I am still losing weight.) We set the prize as a nice dinner of the winning team's choosing to be paid for by the losing team. But I, being a giant dork, insisted that dinner should only be the prize if the losers have to write haikus about the glory of the winners and read them at the dinner. Heh. Hee hee heh. I love haikus. That decision, by the way, prompted this e-mail from my dear friend Peter:

a few words that rhyme with peter

(just in case you need them for your haiku—which technically

shouldn't rhyme, but still . . .)

heater

greeter

beat her

sweeter

defeater

liter

eater

trick-or-treater

neater

seater

meter

teeter

there are many more

you'll have plenty to choose from.

let's be clear—no using

peter's a cheater

who gained a liter cause he's

such a big eater.

beat you to the punch, suckas!

xoxo

p

Oh. Poor Peter. Poor, poor, losing Peter. All that trash talk and no victory to go with it. (And now I'm trash-talking him in a book! So dirty.) It's gonna be sooooo fun tonight to hear him sing my praises in 5-7-5 meter. CAN'T WAIT. Did I mention I'm a big dork?

My point here is, when you choose your prize, it's fine to make it a material thing (dinner, tickets to a show, etc.) but it's surprisingly more effective when it's a thing that can't be bought.

• • • • • • • • • • • • • • • • • • • • • • • • • • • • • • • • • • • • • • • • • • • • •

Playing against your boyfriend/girlfriend/husband/wife?
Here are a few tantalizing prize suggestions
from former players . . .

• • • • • • • • • • • • • • • • • • • • • • • • • • • • • • • • • • • • • • • • • • • • •

- Ten minutes of a serious make-out session every night for a month. "Extras" chosen by winner. (Wink, wink.)
- Every Friday night for a month, the losing partner makes a luxurious bubble bath for the winner and for 20 minutes reads his/her favorite

novel to them as they soak. If there are accents involved, the loser must *do* the accents.

- Loser must call winner every day at noon and say at least five things that genuinely acknowledge your love for the winner and what is so great about them.

You cannot buy your way out of driving carpool for a month.

You cannot buy your way out of doing laundry for a month.

You cannot pay your husband to rub your feet every night for a month.

You cannot pay your friends to write haikus about you. And if you can, your friends are really broke and maybe you should give them some money.

### • • • A Tip from Az • • •

Put a prize up for yourself in addition to the team prize! Make yourself a deal each week: "If I earn at least X amount of points this week, I will buy myself that _____ I've been wanting." It'll give you extra motivation and a weekly bonus for a game well played!

Again, it's not about the prize, really. It's about the spoils of victory and the fun of the game, and, oh, yeah, all the health you'll gain and weight you'll lose along the way. But don't forgo the prize. Because it's important to have an actual thing you're competing for. (In sports psychology, it's widely accepted that a player is motivated best when there are both intrinsic and extrinsic motivating factors. An intrinsic factor is something like a feeling of accomplishment or pride. An extrinsic factor is a prize.)

So pick a thing.

It should be a thing you all want to win.

It should be a thing that will hurt a little to lose.

Like my dinner tonight. Everyone playing can afford the dinner—but the haikus. The haikus are gonna hurt. 'Cause (a) good haikus are hard to write. And (b) they have to be all about the greatness of me (and my team-mate, Adam), which will hurt them to read but please us greatly.

Haikus. Hilarious. Who makes their friends write haikus?? Me. I do.

### If forced poetry is not your thing, here is a brief list of other prize ideas:

- An actual trophy. You can buy one at a party store. Bragging rights galore.
- Tickets to a show (winner's choice).
- Dinner where the winners get to dictate the conversation (e.g.: "Absolutely no politics—I don't care if the debate was last night!"—or "We must discuss *So You Think You Can Dance* for a full half-hour").
- Massages (either the spa kind or the at-home-in-front-of-the-TV-with-your-stinky-feet-in-your-spouse's-lap kind).
- Chores. Office or household or yard work. Any kind of chores.
- Carpool.
- Embarrassing singing telegrams. From the winners to the losers. Paid for by the losers.

The other, slightly less creative, but always effective, way to go is the buy-in. Let's say you have three teams of two players each and everyone kicks in 50 bucks. Now you have a $300 pot that will go to the winning team. Winners get 150 bucks each. Not too shabby. And you can choose the dollar amount based on what the average player can afford. Maybe it's a $10 buy-in. Maybe it's $100. Just remember, it should hurt a little (but not a lot).

Oh, and one final tip: If the prize is money or has monetary value, *everyone must buy in at the beginning of the game.* That way, no one's running around at the end trying to collect cash from sore losers. Trust me. We learned this the hard way.

# Frequently Asked Questions

Q:  Some of my friends make a lot more money than my other friends. How do we choose a prize that satisfies everyone?

A:  It's really important, especially if the prize involves money in any way, that all players are comfortable with what's at stake. You don't ever want financial issues to negatively affect a friendship, so be sensitive to everyone's financial situation when proposing prizes. Consider something inexpensive, but highly victorious, like an evening of karaoke where the winners choose the losers' songs.

Q:  Can we do first, second, and third prizes?

A:  Absolutely, and with a big game going, it's a really fun way to play and keep everyone motivated (especially if there's an early front-runner).

Q:  Can we skip the prize and just play the game?

A:  You can if you want to be stupid and boring your whole life. Hehe. Heh heh heh hee.

Q:  Can the prize be a secret that no one knows until the end?

A:  Ideally, no. The extrinsic motivation factor works best if everyone's in on the prize.

Q:  Can we change the prize halfway through the game and make it bigger?

A:  Hell, yes! Pile it on! (As long as all players agree to the change.)

Q:  Can we change the prize halfway through the game and make it smaller?

A:  No. That's an idea usually proposed by someone who is losing. And that's what we call sour grapes.

# GET A PEN!

List a few of your own ideas for prizes. And if you're feeling really punchy, try writing them as a haiku. It's surprisingly hard . . .

_____

_____

_____

_____

_____

_____

_____

_____

_____

_____

_____

_____

_____

_____

_____

By the way, here was Peter's haiku from dinner . . .

_Adam drags Krista_
_across the finish line. What_
_hollow victory._

(Hmm. Mean. He got the last word after all . . .)

Chapter 6

# THE HONOR SYSTEM

## (Or, No, French Fries REALLY Don't Count as a Vegetable.)

One of the truest tests of integrity is its blunt
refusal to be compromised.

—*Chinua Achebe*

When I was five years old, I developed a system for shoplifting. My girlfriend Gina and I would pull a little red wagon around our Venice Beach neighborhood. We would tuck our favorite stuffed animals into the wagon and cover them with a blanket, telling amused passersby that they were taking a nap. Then we would pull said blanket-covered wagon into the corner convenience store and when no one was looking, we'd tuck a bunch of candy under the blanket along with the sleeping stuffed animals, and then take off and binge in the alley behind the store.

Five years old.

True story.

When I was fifteen years old, I was still using a version of this system when I was finally arrested for shoplifting. My girlfriend Jamille and I would skip school and go to the mall. We would bring empty shopping bags and stuff our winter coats into them. Then we would walk into stores like The Gap and The Limited and, in the dressing room, we'd pull the coats out, stuff the bags full of unpurchased clothes, and then leave the store, still carrying full shopping bags, but now wearing our winter coats.

By the time we got busted—and by busted, I mean, *chased through the mall* by a small Asian woman yelling "STOP! THIEF!"—we had *thousands of dollars* of stolen clothes in our closets. This was the end of my shoplifting career. The arrest, the handcuffs, going to court, and having to see a probation officer every week for six months . . . the whole thing scared me straight.

But I still have a sneaky mind. I'm a Scorpio, after all. A Scorpio from a fucked up family. In my early twenties, when I decided to quit drinking and teach myself how to become a grown-up, I had to learn how not to lie, cheat, or steal. I figured out with the guidance of some really great mentors that lying, cheating, and stealing were the quickest ways to an untrusting mind and an unhappy life. Changing wasn't easy. I had to practice being an honest person the way a kid has to practice riding a bike. I was so used to lying—not crazy, pathological lying, but "what lie can I tell to avoid getting in trouble?" lying. I told habitual lies like, "I'm sorry I'm late, the traffic was terrible" when the truth was I just left too late to get there on time. Constant little corruptions that ate away at my soul.

So I was instructed to try to live an honest life one lie at a time. Every time I would hear a lie come out of my mouth, I would correct it. I would literally say, "I'm sorry, I just totally lied. There wasn't much traffic; I just left late. Sorry." If I didn't catch the lie in the moment, I would call later and amend it. Extreme? Maybe. But I was trying to undo a twenty-year habit of unconscious lying—it required extreme measures.

And eventually, I succeeded. I very rarely lie anymore and when I do, I literally feel it in my body. It's like foreign matter in my gut—like a burning, tingling, disturbing feeling that probably has something to do with adrenaline but is terribly uncomfortable for me until I catch the lie and make amends. And I never steal. I won't even do little things like sneak into a movie theater to catch a second movie without going out to the ticket booth and buying another ticket. Not because I think I'm all superior, but because any kind of lying and stealing leads me down a path of more of the same. Scorpio mind.

I'm sharing this with you, a total stranger, because it's important to me that you understand that the integrity aspect of this game is not always easy for me. My sneaky mind can come up with A THOUSAND WAYS to bend the rules. Right now, I'm playing the game and the bad habit I gave up is complacency. I stated to my team that that means I'm doing a minimum of three yogic Sun Salutations every day. Last night, I was on my way to bed when I realized I had forgotten to do my yoga. My brain instantly went like this: *Yeah, but you gave up complacency. And you paced in the writer's room today. You probably clocked a mile. That's not complacent. So you can skip the yoga and not lose your points.* Which is a total and complete cheat. It's a balls-out lie—but I can make a balls-out lie sound *really good* if I put my mind to it. I gave myself a little talking-to. It sounded like this: *Do the yoga or lose the points. These are your only options, Psycho.* I did the yoga. And you know what? I figured out that there's a reason it's called Sun Salutation. It's highly energizing. Not a great thing right before bed. And now I know. It took me forever to fall asleep—but I didn't lose my points.

*I have young children and would prefer they don't grow up sounding like truckers, so for my bad habit, I gave up the word "fuck." It proved very hard. The very first day, within half an hour of waking up, I said "fuck." Then I thought FUCK, I just said "fuck." Then I thought, this wasn't very fair, I just woke up, my brain isn't even fully awake, I haven't even had my coffee, how can I be held responsible? When filling out my score for the day, I ultimately didn't give myself the points for my bad habit. With great resolve I told myself I would do better tomorrow. The next day came and then FUCK flew out of my mouth. Really? How could this happen? As I thought about it, I just realized how present I had to be in every moment of my life. The rest of the week I earned my points.*

—Jana, 40

Here's another, far more painful, example. In my one-on-one game with Az, we were neck-and-neck for three weeks—both pulling down perfect scores. And then in week four, I was super tired one day and I was trying not to drink coffee 'cause I was fighting off a cold and coffee tends to make me lose the fight and so I walked over to the commissary and I bought an iced tea/lemonade, and I drank the whole thing before I realized there was sugar and high-fructose corn sweetener in the lemonade. It was basically soda. Which is not a game-sanctioned food. I didn't even have half lemonade, half iced tea. I had *mostly* iced tea and probably 40 calories of lemonade.

EVERYTHING IN ME wanted to ignore it, or justify it somehow. My brain went CRAZY. *Could it be my meal off? No, because I already had my meal off. Could it be my hundred calories of anything? No, I already had those today. But it wasn't really a treat! It wasn't intentional! It was a mistake! I wasn't thinking! I can't be penalized for being TIRED, for God's sake. I'm a mom. My kid wakes me up all the time. Plus I'm getting sick. I'm soooo tired. Of course I wasn't thinking clearly. I should not be docked for this. Forget it. I just won't even mention it. Stupid lemonade. Whatever.* And then it tortured me for days. And when it came time to turn in our score sheets to each other, I just couldn't live with it. It was a freaking snacking penalty.

Why, you say? Why, when it was an *honest mistake*, should I lose the game over it?

Because once my husband unthinkingly popped some blueberries in his mouth and he had to take a snacking penalty for it. And when he asked me why, I said, "Because the game is designed to make us think BE-FORE we toss calories into our mouths." Unconscious eating is a serious culprit in a lot of people's weight gain. And if you have to take a penalty for "not thinking" enough times, eventually, you will start to think before you eat.

You know what Az and I had bet? A new iPhone. And you KNOW I'm still pissed. I'm convinced that sometimes he calls me on it for no good reason. Juuuuust to rub it in. Aussie bastard.

*My first point-loss was on day one of my first game. I absently pulled a half-piece of carrot from my bag and ate it as I walked to the car, without even noticing until I swallowed it. Now, this was before the 100-calorie rule. A half of a piece of carrot. This was going to cost me my first point in this game? And, right off the bat, I decided not to say anything, to let it slide: That didn't count. It was absent-mindedness. It's not like it was a Snickers! It was a carrot! Less than a carrot! The game is not anti-carrot! Do-over!*

*And then I realized if I was going to play, then it did count—it had to count—because it's not the eating of carrots that I'm trying to fight, it's the absent-mindedness. It's the habit of noticing when I'm putting food in my mouth that I needed to develop. So I told someone about it right away, to shut up the devil on my shoulder. And, it turns out it was the last time I ever lost points for absent-minded eating.*

—Bill, 40

This entire game is about integrity. It's the one key ingredient you cannot play without. When I invited one of my coworkers to play, she said, "Wait—it's an honor system thing? No way, I know myself, I'll just cheat." And I loved her for that. I loved her, ironically, for her honesty. You gotta know yourself. You gotta know if you can keep it honest. Because this game is played with your friends and family and colleagues. And even though it's a game, when you put money or a prize on the line—not to mention the all-important bragging rights—people take it seriously. Once, my friend Greg had to take a snacking penalty for a Tic Tac. A TIC TAC. The "One-Calorie Breath Mint." Why? Because someone on an opposing team saw him eat it. And this was before we added the 100-calories-of-whatever rule. And the person on the opposing team sent all the players of that very big game this e-mail:

> I saw Greg eating a Tic Tac. If he comes up with a perfect score this week, we will all know he's a big fat cheater.

And who wants to be known as a big fat cheater? No one. That's who.

● ● ● ● ● ● ● ● ● ● ● ● ● ● ● ● ● ● ● ● ● ● ● ● ● ● ● ● ● ● ● ● ● ● ● ● ● ● ● ● ● ● ● ● ●

## A word from Heide Banks on Integrity

*Most people don't understand what integrity really means. It is not about doing things that are right/wrong or good/bad but rather keeping your word with yourself, 100 percent. You decide to do something, agree to do it 100 percent and you stop weighing options from that moment forward. To paraphrase John-Roger, doing anything at the 99-percent level is a bitch; move to 100 percent and everything becomes a breeze.*

*Living outside of personal integrity has some very real consequences. Even the smallest of lies takes energy—both mental and physical—to maintain. This is also why when you keep your agreements, especially to yourself, you will often feel a surge of energy.*

*I think you have to start with the assumption that we are all very good at lying to ourselves, and unless we keep an antidote on hand that counteracts our ability to do this, we will fail at whatever we attempt. That magic pill is integrity, complete, unfettered, 100 percent integrity.*

*Don't be surprised to find other areas of your life start to change as a direct result of your new commitment to yourself. Friends and relationships that supported and perhaps even encouraged your breaking agreements may drop away, and don't be surprised if you have more time and energy on your hands. Use this time to reward yourself with nurturing activities and welcome in new relationships . . . especially the one you are creating with yourself, your authentic self.*

*There is another benefit, perhaps even more important than weight loss, that we encounter when we stop lying to ourselves and demand 100 percent self-integrity. We finally come in touch with the emotional pain we have been pushing down with food and other distractions, and now have the ability to heal and transform that pain into joy and fulfillment.*

*—Heide Banks, coach, psychotherapist, and author*
*www.heidebanks.com*

• • • • • • • • • • • • • • • • • • • • • • • • • • • • • • • •

Play.

Play all out.

There is no benefit for you in cheating at this game. No benefit for you and no benefit for your waistline. One of the main objects of the game is to take weight off. Guilt is a mental and emotional weight, so lying entirely defeats the purpose. (And may lead to sleeplessness, which will lose you sleep points, and may find you raiding the fridge at 3 a.m., which will lose you snacking points. See? Vicious cycle.)

## • • • A Tip from Az • • •

If you are truly not sure about your score—like, say, you ate a meal that you think maybe shouldn't be sanctioned—take it in your mind to the most incorruptible person you can think of. Maybe it's your mum, or Buddha or Jesus or the Dalai Lama or Nelson Mandela or Mother Teresa. Ask yourself how they would score themselves in this situation. Usually, this will give you your answer. Because usually, if you're not sure, it's because you've lost points and you're looking for a way out of it. But if, after practicing this exercise, you're still not sure, then take it to an opponent (not a teammate!) and ask him or her to be the judge. (And ideally, it should not be an opponent who is married to you and can be made to suffer for his or her answer. If it is, get a second opinion!)

It all comes down to this: When I play honestly, I feel tremendous pride when I have a high-scoring week because it's HARD to get a high-scoring week in this game. It requires huge effort for most of us and a huge commitment to change. And the pride of victory leads to further commitment to change.

And when my scores slip, I always learn something about myself. Well, first, I watch my brain try to formulate the lie. But then I learn something about myself. Whether I lost points because I wasn't paying attention or because I was doing some emotional eating, or because I stayed up too late composing e-mails to a crazy friend (Hey! Look at that! I prioritized her crazy over my own health!) I always learn something. Of course, learning something is one thing. Facing my team, and telling them I let them down, is always another. That part is hard. That part is why it's sometimes VERY tempting to lie. But when you tell the truth, you not only get to learn about yourself, you get to learn something about your friends.

Guys . . . I think I have to drop out. As you know, I'm launching my new business and I can't do the work till the baby goes to sleep which means I can't get 7 hours of sleep a night and get done what needs to be done. It's actually humanly impossible. And I have deadlines I have to meet. And I can't stand that I keep losing sleep points for you guys. Can I play next time? I'm so sorry.

Brooke

Brookie,

You need this game right now. If you aren't getting enough sleep, you need to be eating well and drinking enough water and getting a little exercise. So even if you lose sleep points every night, we want you to keep playing. Besides, you know the guys' team is losing points like crazy. I heard Greg was eating Tic Tacs. Don't drop out!

xoxo,

Us

The fact here is that Brooke was telling the truth and her team knew it. And so she got the support she needed to prioritize her health to the best of her current ability. Which is what the game is all about.

So if you slip, face your team, tell them what happened—and try to do it on the day you slip rather than at the end of the week. That way, you will get support throughout the week so it's less likely to happen again. Of course, sometimes the support looks more like this:

Dude. I ate onion rings last night. Oops.

Joe

You are a lazy bastard. I am not about to lose to a bunch of chicks. So stop losing us points or I will kick your fat ass the next time I see you.

Jake

Now, Joe was indeed being a lazy bastard. But at least he was an *honest* lazy bastard. He could've just lied. You could always just lie. But don't do it. The gain is simply not worth the loss. Seriously. Lie on your scores and the next thing you know the lady from the Jade Pagoda could be chasing you through the mall yelling, "Stop! Thief!" Which makes for a great story eventually, but at the time? No fun at all.

# Frequently Asked Questions

Q: What should I do if I think an opponent is lying every week to make his or her points?

A: Keep your own scores honest, play all out anyway, and don't play with the lying fuck next time. Maybe put a side bet on the table with one of your opponents or a teammate or even with yourself— that way you stay motivated to keep your scores honest and high. Remember, the liar has to live with himself. So you don't need to take revenge, because a liar's miserable mind is its own revenge.

Q: I don't trust anyone. How can I possibly play this game?

A: Umm . . . maybe you should play by yourself and make a weekly appointment with a good therapist to work on your trust issues? Seriously, not trusting anyone is no way to go through life.

Q: What if I suspect my own teammate of lying?

A: Talk to them. Tell them that because you are a true friend, you would not have them sacrifice their soul for a winning score. Also, consider a group weigh-in each week. You can't confirm all their scores with the weigh in, but you can be sure that they are at least doing the work to lose the weight, and thereby gaining some health benefits. Finally, use the power of example. Often, a liar lies because they're desperate to present a perfect face to the world. If you lose points, call your friend and tell on yourself. Show them that it's okay to not look perfect all the time.

Q: Sometimes I lie about doing 20 minutes of exercise one day, but I do 40 minutes the next, that's okay? Right?

A: No! No lying!! The rules are called rules for a reason. And they are all designed with your very best health in mind.

Q: Can our team make up a rule that if a team member makes an *honest* mistake, they get to be forgiven one time without a penalty?

A:   No. They can and should be forgiven. But they have to take the point penalty. *The goal here is not a perfect score at any cost. The goal is the best score you can honestly accomplish.* The slips teach you about yourself, your life, your health habits, and where you need to start to pay more attention. Letting yourself off the hook is actually selling yourself short. Don't do it!

Q:   What if I eat something that I think is sanctioned and then find out it was cooked in butter or something unsanctioned? Do I lose the points?

A:   Before I started playing this game, I thought crab cakes were a healthy choice at a restaurant. Crab is relatively low-calorie and high-protein and it's a small portion, right? So I ordered them and I ate them and they were delicious. And then, out of curiosity, I typed them into the calorie-counting Web site and I was, like, yay! Only 400 calories! And then I realized it was 400 calories per crab cake. And I had eaten two. 800 calories—as an appetizer. Clearly, I was not understanding the ingredients. Clearly they are full of butter and mayonnaise, which I now understand but truly did not before. I lost points—but I learned something. If you ate something without knowing how it was cooked, you are probably in the habit of eating things without knowing how they're cooked, which is probably a big part of why you have weight you want to lose. So yes, you lose the points. But the good news is you probably won't make that mistake again.

Q:   Have you ever had a situation where you felt you were losing points unfairly?

A:   Yes. When my daughter was sick with a terrible cold and she was up every fifteen minutes all night nursing. By 2 a.m., having not slept a wink, I was STARVING to death because making breast milk requires calorie intake, so I ate a banana and took a snacking penalty. The next day, I told Az about it, and he said hell no, that should not be a penalty. You prioritized your health and the health of your daughter. So we took it to a vote—all the players on all teams had to vote. And it was voted that I should not lose the points. BUT! This kind of circumstance is rare. If you have a similar situation—*don't just assume it's not a penalty!* Take the penalty and then put it to a vote. A vote keeps you honest. And when voting, everyone should keep in mind that the spirit of the game is to support your teammates and opponents in their pursuit of health. Don't be an asshole and vote against anyone just because you want them to lose the points. (That's a great rule for life in general: Don't be an asshole.) That said, if you lose the vote, take the penalty and do not be bitter. As with any sport, if you think the ref made a bad call, you still have to play the game in the spirit of good sportsmanship. Or you can go all John McEnroe on their asses. Which is always fun to watch.

• • • • • • • • • • • • • • • • • • • • • • • • • • • • • • • • • • • • • • •

## Play by the Rules

• • • • • • • • • • • • • • • • • • • • • • • • • • • • • • • • • • • • • • •

- Keep your own score with absolute integrity.
- If you're not sure about a rule, look it up in this book; don't just assume.
- If you think you may have lost points, but aren't sure, you probably lost points; but if you're really not sure, run it past an opponent.
- Consider weekly group weigh-ins to keep yourselves honest (and to add fun and camaraderie to the game).
- Never prioritize how you "look" over how you feel. Lying will make you feel like crap. Don't do it.

## Mandy Collins, *lost 55 pounds*

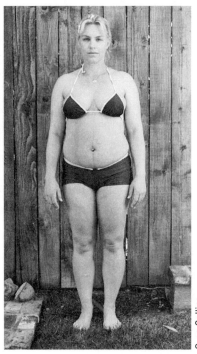 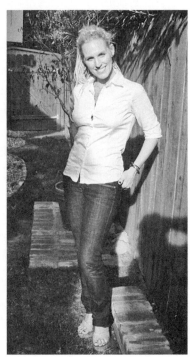

Greg Collins                                          Greg Collins

While pregnant with my third child, I gained more than seventy pounds. I'm naturally slim, and I knew I needed some extra weight to sustain a healthy pregnancy—but this got a little out of hand! After my daughter was born, I was a little overwhelmed by the uphill battle I saw in the mirror each morning. The game gave me the added incentive (not to mention the hilarious daily trash-talk e-mails) I needed to do the work to take the weight off. I played several games, and kept up the eating and exercise plan between games and eventually, came to look like myself again! (Chasing my three-year-old twin boys around all day helped too!) I love the game—I love the healthy competition, the supportive community, and I love what it did for my body and for my spirit!

Mandy Collins, 37

# Chapter 7

# THE WEIGH-IN

## (Or, You're Kidding, Right? You Want Me to Buy a Scale? SERIOUSLY???)

What kind of scale compares the weight of two beauties, the gravity of duties, or the ground speed of joy? Tell me, what kind of gauge can quantify elation? What kind of equation could I possibly employ?

—*Ani DiFranco*

**The Rule:** Weigh yourself on the Monday morning you start the game, within 10 minutes of waking. Then, weigh in once a week on the morning of your day off. Weigh yourself Saturday morning if Saturday will be your day off. Weigh yourself Sunday morning if Sunday will be your day off. (The point is, you don't want to weigh in the morning AFTER your day off!)

Each week, you must lose 1 percent of your body weight to earn a bonus that equals 20 percent of your points scored for the week.

**Calculations:** Your weight x .01 = The number of pounds you must lose to earn your bonus points

Your points scored for the week x .2 = Your bonus points if you make weight!

If in any given week you do not earn your weight-loss bonus (lose 1 percent of your body weight), you lose your alcohol privilege on both your free day and during your meal off *for the rest of the game*.

**Note:** If weight loss is not a goal, you can set yourself a fitness goal instead.

**Penalty:** DO NOT WEIGH YOURSELF MORE THAN ONCE A DAY. IF YOU DO, YOU LOSE A POINT EACH EXTRA TIME YOU GET ON THE SCALE!

**Believe me, Az** and I spent a looooot of time discussing and debating whether or not to include this rule. The arguments went something like this:

**Me:** No way. No way are we asking women or men or anyone to weigh in every week. Scales suck. Scales are mean. People hate scales.

**Az:** The game is played on an honor system and it's not an exact science.

How else can we be sure people are (a) not cheating and (b) playing correctly for their maximum health benefit?

**Me:** Did I mention how much scales suck?

**Az:** Do you have a better idea?

**Me:** (silence)

**Az:** The scale's important. It's about making sure people are on the right track. It's a feedback tool. All it's letting us know is whether we've eaten the right amount of food or too much or too little. It's one thing to be eating healthy, but if you're eating too much of healthy then you will put on weight, which is not healthy. I know a lot of people who only eat organic health foods and their body is a temple, but they are thirty pounds overweight. These are the people who come to me and say "What the fuck, man? I'm the healthiest person I know!" The fact is they're eating too much of a good thing, and if they'd gotten on the scale when they were five pounds overweight instead of thirty, they could have made changes sooner. We have to include a weigh-in.

**Me:** (silence)

**Az:** Krista? You still there?

**Me:** Shut up, you Aussie bitch.

If your reaction here is *no way in hell am I getting on a scale because scales make me crazy and make me want to cry and make me want to throw them across the room,* believe me, I relate. But in the end, I gave in to Az on this one not only because I didn't have a better idea about how to help you confirm that you're playing right, but because I didn't weigh myself for many, many years and that was a big part of what allowed me to get so heavy.

I gave up scales for a good reason. I gave up scales because I tend to go to extremes, and scales in my bathroom, historically, got way too much play. Like, *I'm not really this heavy, right? This has to be some kind of mistake. This thing must be broken. Hmmmm, if I weigh myself after I pee, will I lose a pound? What about after I shower? Could I scrub off a pound or two of dirt? What about after I sweat?* Worse than that, the number on the scale in the morning would dictate my mood for the entire day. I would fixate and obsess and feel powerless and then fixate and obsess some more.

So I got rid of the scale. And I never once missed it. I didn't miss it to an extreme. I didn't miss it so much, I became obese and didn't notice.

So when Az asked me to get a scale for the game, I had a strong reaction, somewhere between fear and loathing. And I ranted at him for a while about how crazy I am and how crazy having a scale in the house would make me. And then he cocked his head at me and said, "Are you sure you're still that kind of crazy? You don't strike me that way. Maybe you could just get a scale and keep it in the closet and weigh yourself once a week."

Honestly, it hadn't even occurred to me. It hadn't occurred to me that when I was last making myself crazy with a scale I was a teenager. And that maybe now I have grown and changed and healed enough to have some moderation, to have all the information without using it to torture myself all day every day, to not have my day defined and shaped by the number staring up at me from between my toes each morning.

*I lost eight pounds playing the game but more important I can fit into my pants again (with no muffin top!). I really loved all that I learned about food. It is amazing what junk we put into our bodies that should not even be called food. I feel I learned how to respect myself and my body while I was playing the game. Krista and Az are geniuses. They should win a Nobel Peace Prize or an Academy Award for all the work they do. I want to be just like them. (Did I go too far?)*

*—Michael, 36*

I've said it before and I'll say it again: Having all the information is empowering. And weighing yourself once a week is how you get all the information. What do I mean by that? Well, the first week he played this game, my husband *gained weight.* Why? He wasn't paying that much attention when Az explained the rules and important little things like portion sizing. So he went from three relatively large meals a day to five relatively large meals a day. Had he not weighed in, he might have stayed on that path and gotten the opposite result that anyone is hoping for. Instead, he got on the scale at the end of the week and went, *WTF?* And Az said,

"Let's have a look at what you're eating." Kevin then went on to steadily lose twenty pounds.

So let's just decide right now that we're not going to make this a whole big emotional thing. Let's just let it be a tool—one tool in a big toolbox of health. Just get up, pee, and then get on the scale. Naked. And remember, the number on the scale is just a starting point. A fact. A number. It's a number just like the number in your car that tells you how fast you are going. It's not a giant sign that says "you're a big fat-ass loser." So for the length of the game, take the emotion out of the number. For four weeks, give up making that number mean something bad about you. The number on the scale tells you where you are today and in four weeks it will tell you how far you have come.

To help, we've implemented a penalty for getting on the scale more than once a day. This is designed to help you let go of the unhealthy obsessing and embrace the health of having all the information!

## Step Up Your Game!

Some tips for making friends with your scale.

- Paste a happy picture on your scale. Maybe a picture of your kid or your spouse or your pet smiling or making a funny face. Let the picture remind you that (a) you have a great reason to get healthy and (b) you should be smiling too because the number on the scale is just a number. It does not quantify *you*.
- Weigh yourself either once every morning or once every week. The rest of the time, keep the scale out of sight, in a closet or under your sink.
- If two members of your household are playing, surprise each other by redecorating the scale every day or two! Funny pictures of your family one day. Crazy porn the next. Keep each other guessing and keep yourselves laughing.

Believe it or not, I have come to look forward to weighing in each week that I'm playing the game. Because every week I've played but two, I've lost weight. I've done it consciously, I've done it healthily, and I've done it without obsessing or fixating. And that is such a good feeling.

## • • • A Tip from Az • • •

If you have no need or desire to lose weight and are hoping instead to firm or bulk up, set yourself a fitness goal as a way of earning your bonus points. How would that work? Something like this: Do a HIIT workout on Monday. (See Chapter 9, Exercise.) If you do it on a stationary bike, and the highest you can go is, say, level 6, then set yourself a goal of reaching level 7 by Sunday. If you do it, you get your bonus points. The key here, as with every other aspect of this game, is *complete integrity.* Ride as hard as you can on Monday. And then train like hell to beat yourself a week later. If you don't do it, you don't get the bonus points! You can also set yourself a distance goal (if you can run only five miles on Monday, you want to be able to run five and half by Saturday). Or a weightlifting goal (set yourself a goal weight) . . . You get the idea. But before you make this decision, keep in mind that if you have unwanted fat anywhere on your body, you have to lose weight to get rid of it. YOU CANNOT TURN FAT INTO MUSCLE. You have to lose the fat (lose the weight) and then build muscle in its place!

## Frequently Asked Questions

Q: I have my period/am constipated/am bloated. I think that's why I didn't lose weight. What do I do?

A: See Chapter 16, Troubleshooting.

Q: Should I weigh in every day or just once a week?

A:     Studies show that dieters who weigh themselves every day lose up
       to twice as much weight as dieters who weigh in once a week. So I
       weigh myself every day. It keeps me honest and motivated. But it's
       really up to you.

Q:     Can I get some of my points if I lost .99 percent of my weight?
A:     No. Sorry. We gotta keep the rule clean and clear. But if you lost
       .99 percent of your weight, you rock and you know it. That's your
       reward.

Q:     Our team wants to reward any kind of weight loss even if it's not 1
       percent. Suggestions? Can we make up our own point system?
A:     Truly, you can do whatever you want as long as your whole team
       and all of your opponents agree. We find the game to be most ef-
       fective when played by our rules, but we respect your desire to do
       your thing. Just make sure you're all agreed as to what your thing
       is! (FYI: The reason we chose 1 percent is that it levels the playing
       field—often a heavier person will lose weight more quickly than a
       lighter person.)

Q:     Why do I have to lose my alcohol for the entire game? I'd rather
       lose my 100 free calories or my meal off. Can I trade?
A:     No. This isn't meant to punish you. It really is because alcohol can
       slow the body's ability to burn fat by a whopping 73 percent!! It is
       a major reason why people fail to lose weight on diets. Again, not
       a punishment—just an effort to help you step up your game and
       meet your fitness goals. Really. Truly. Love ya. Mean it.

Q:     Does it matter what kind of scale I use? Is electronic better?
A:     Just use the same scale at the same time of day every week.

Q:     To make things fair, shouldn't we all be using the same kind
       of scale on our teams? It seems easier to cheat with those dial
       scales.
A:     Nobody is cheating. We all have integrity. PLEASE please please,

let's all play with integrity! But if you're concerned, have a group weigh in!

Q:  When I first started the game, I liked the scale because I kept losing weight. But now I've hit a plateau and I HATE it. It depresses me when I start to walk toward the scale for weigh in. I don't want to feel this way. Any suggestions?

A:  Yes. Step up your exercise and/or cut back your calories. Then do this exercise . . .

## GET A PEN!

On the following lines, list ten great things about you that have nothing to do with the number on the scale. Then read them aloud to yourself. This describes you. The number on the scale does not!

_____

_____

_____

_____

_____

_____

_____

_____

_____

_____

_____

_____

_____

_____

_____

_____

● ● ● ● ● ● ● ● ● ● ● ● ● ● ● ● ● ● ● ● ● ● ● ● ● ● ● ● ● ● ● ● ● ● ● ● ● ● ● ● ● ●

## Play by the Rules

● ● ● ● ● ● ● ● ● ● ● ● ● ● ● ● ● ● ● ● ● ● ● ● ● ● ● ● ● ● ● ● ● ● ● ● ● ● ● ● ●

- Weigh yourself on the morning you start the game, within 10 minutes of waking.
- Once a week, weigh yourself the morning of your day off.
- Each week you must lose 1 percent of your body weight to earn a bonus that equals 20 percent of your points scored for the week.
- If you do not earn your weight-loss bonus you must give up drinking alcohol for the remainder of the game.
- Remember that the weigh-in is designed to be a feedback tool that helps you see your progress and educates you as to where you may need to make some adjustments.
- If you weigh yourself more than once a day, you lose one point for every extra time you get on the scale.
- Remember that the number on the scale is just a number. It empowers you by giving you all the information you need to succeed in meeting your fitness goals.
- For the length of the game, try taking the emotion out of the number on the scale. Give up making that number mean anything bad about you.
- Studies have shown that those who weigh themselves daily have more success with weight loss.
- If you really hate your scale, try decorating it with something that makes you happy every time you see it.

# Chapter 8

# FOOD

### (Or, Why French Fries Don't Count as a Vegetable.)

My doctor told me to stop having
intimate dinners for four;
unless there are three other people.

—*Orson Welles*

**The Rule**: Eat five small meals a day. Each meal should include a combination of lean protein, healthy fats, carbohydrates like whole grains and fruit, and/or vegetables. Meals must be no fewer than two and no more than four hours apart. Meals must contain none of the F.L.A.B.B. foods you will find listed in this chapter. Each fully sanctioned meal is worth 6 points for a total of 30 possible meal points a day.

**The Exception**: Each day, in addition to your five meals, you may consume up to 100 calories of whatever you want (including the F.L.A.B.B. foods on the list, but *not* including alcohol, soda, or diet soda).

**Note**: Between meals, you may snack on cucumbers and celery without penalty.

**Penalty**: If you eat anything between meals besides cucumbers and celery, you must deduct a 10-point snacking penalty. You must include veggies in at least two of your meals or you will not recieve your meal points for those meals.

**When my daughter** was six weeks old, my sister and her family came from New York to visit for five wonderful days. I was on maternity leave and my husband and I were hunkered down in new baby bliss. (Except that one time she decided to poo while we were all in the bathtub together. That was slightly less than blissful.) We had the intoxicating love of new parenthood, a lot of doting and helpful friends and family to help, and tons of time—the most precious commodity and the one I hadn't had enough of in years. It was the happiest time of my life so far and my sister's visit was the icing on the happy cake. We went out to breakfast and lunch every day and ordered dinner in and lounged around the house ogling the baby and making those cooing baby-talk noises that all twentysomethings swear to God they will never make.

When my sister went back to New York after five days, she sent me this e-mail:

> We had the best time ever! I love Coco soooooo much I want to eat her. But I probably shouldn't since I got on my scale this morning and saw that I GAINED FOUR POUNDS. Four pounds in five days! All that vacation eating was fun—but daaaaamn, now I gotta hit the gym. No Coco eating for me. Miss you!
>
> Kaisteroni

Most pressingly, Kaisteroni is a name I affectionately call my sister— a combination of Kaili, sister, and macaroni-head. I have no idea why macaroni-head. Anyway, I wrote her back an e-mail that went something like this . . .

> Dude. Scales are stupid. And depending on what time of day you weigh yourself, they change. There's no way you gained four pounds.

And then she wrote me back . . .

> Dudette. I gained four pounds. For reals. On my way to gym now. Ugh.
>
> xxooo

This was just a casual e-mail exchange for my sister, but for me it was a huge wake-up call. *Kaili gained four pounds in five days by eating what I was eating every day.* This was not "vacation eating" for me. This was my habitual, daily diet. Omelets and potatoes and toast for breakfast. Tuna melts for lunch. Pasta and bread and copious crab cake–like appetizers for dinner. And then, dessert. Every day.

> *Here's the thing—I don't cook. I'm bad at it, I hate grocery stores, I would much rather order in every meal. But the game taught me really great ways to keep food in the house, to take care of myself (like a*

*grown-up) and that's when the weight came off. It wasn't that hard, I just needed some motivation—and the game has motivation in SPADES.*

—Pete, 38

You see, I had been told that breastfeeding burns, like, 500 extra calories a day (and it does). And I can tell you for certain that breastfeeding makes you extra hungry. And I was walking to breakfast every morning. Walking in Los Angeles! Pushing a baby stroller! Almost a mile each way! I thought for sure that balanced any *extra* extra calories I had been eating. Plus, twenty-five pounds of my pregnancy weight had dropped off in the first two weeks after my baby was born, so I figured it would kinda just keep going that way. But when I went to my six-week checkup post-baby, *I had not lost any more weight. None. In a month.* And I couldn't figure out why—until I got that e-mail from my sister.

I am not dumb. And I am a person who has something of a lifelong "issue" with food and weight. So I did have a basic understanding of the "calories in vs. calories burned" concept. But because it had been a long, long time since I had bothered reading calorie contents or really even thinking about them besides the most basic "French fries, I should probably pass on those," what I didn't have was an understanding of just how many calories were in the foods I was casually eating each day. I would usually skip the fries that came with the tuna melt, yeah. But do you know how many calories are in your average tuna melt?? It's two large pieces of bread—about 300 calories. Plus several teaspoons of oil or butter—another 300 or more. Plus cheese—probably about 300 calories' worth. Plus fish—hey, only 200 calories! Plus the mayonnaise that's mixed with the fish—I'm estimating low at 200. That's 1,300 calories. Which is well over half of the calories that almost anyone should be consuming in a day. And that was just my *lunch.*

You're panicking now because I'm talking about calories. I get that. You're having flashbacks to the eighties: calorie counting, Jane Fonda in a leotard, Richard Simmons in a unitard. But allow me to point out that *the country was skinnier in the eighties.* We didn't become morbidly obese as a nation until we threw out calorie counting for fad ideas like counting fat grams. (*Hey! Pasta's fat free! I'll eat a pound!*) That said, if you are still panicking, let me assure you that the game does not require you to count calories. But we *really* encourage you to understand the basic concept!

- - - - - - - - - - - - - - - - - - - - - - - - - - - - - - - - - - - - - - - - - - - -
## Step Up Your Game!
- - - - - - - - - - - - - - - - - - - - - - - - - - - - - - - - - - - - - - - - - - - -

Know this: There is only one way to lose weight. *You must burn more energy than you consume.* That's it! End of story.

YOU MUST BURN MORE ENERGY THAN YOU CONSUME!

Please note that this is completely different from "eating less and exercising more," because you can eat an amount of food that is *less* than what you were eating previously and still be *consuming more energy,* depending on your food choices. You can also exercise for longer than you have before and still be *burning less energy* than you have in the past, depending on your choice of exercise.

So to step up your game, go to www.thegameondiet.com and enter your height, weight, and age. The Web site will do a quick and free calculation for you and tell you how many calories you should be eating each day. (You can also have a trainer at your gym help you come to this number—but he or she will want to pinch your back fat to get it!) Once you have this figure, you will be truly armed with *all the information you need* to lose weight and keep it off! You can then read the calorie content on the foods you're choosing (or you can enter the foods you're choosing into our Web site and we'll let you know the calorie content). This will help you when the game is over, and for the rest of your life, to truly understand when you gain weight WHY you gained weight (and how to lose it).

## • • • A Tip from Az • • •

Before the low-carb diet became such a huge dieting fad, it was known for years as the bodybuilders diet. It seems that some capitalizing people took note of the amazing results that bodybuilders get before going into competition—in particular, with minimizing their body fat.

But it's important that you understand that bodybuilders go on this type of diet for a very short time (just for their "rip up phase" before a competition) and they do it *knowing full well* that as soon as the competition is over they will go back to a healthier, more sustainable way of eating and they will gain weight back.

So when you choose a diet that is all protein and fats and very low carb, you have to realize that the choice you are making is *not sustainable,* because your body is *not getting all the nutrients it needs.* You might get decent results while you are on the diet, but when you go off the diet you will gain weight back and find yourself in the miserable phenomenon known as yo-yo dieting. So if you've ultimately "failed" on one of these diets, don't look at yourself and say "if only I had more discipline . . ." It is not you, it's the diet!

Better to have a healthy blend of all nutrients—including carbs. Goodbye, bacon. Hello, potato!

The food plan I'm about to lay out for you is nothing new. We're simply asking you to eat in the way that nutritionists across the globe now understand to be the healthiest way to lose weight. And it's actually quite simple, but that doesn't make it *easy.*

It's not easy at first because, for most of us, it's new. We are asking you to eat five meals a day when most of us, for most of our lives, have been eating three. (Many dieters, for much of their lives, have been eating even fewer.) So not only is this a change (and man, do I resist change), but five small meals requires more thought and more preparation than three.

*Losing weight was the easy part. It was committing to an eating regi-*
*men that required me to be prepared to eat every two to three hours*
*that was difficult. But to my amazement, I found that other areas of my*
*chaotic, fly-by-the-seat-of-my-pants work/lifestyle became more orga-*
*nized and manageable, achievable even, as I created order around*
*eating. Even my finances showed improvement. And mood swings I*
*used to attribute to an artist's temperament proved to just be low blood*
*sugar. So much for the portrait of the artist. Consistent food and sleep,*
*the new miracle drugs.*

*—Anselm, 36*

We are also giving you a list of F.L.A.B.B. foods. Also known as "Fat-loading and Belly-bloating foods." Hee. Avoiding these foods—a lot of the foods we've all been eating habitually for years—takes extra thought at mealtime. Five mealtimes a day. And most of us really don't want to spend any more time thinking about food than we already do. Except . . .

We say we don't want to have to think about food that much and then we *obsess* about our bodies. We obsess and we obsess *powerlessly.* I swear to you, that by having all the information—by truly understanding how my metabolism works and what is in the foods I choose, I end up thinking about it all *much less.* Because when I wake up in the morning and I put on my jeans and they don't fit and I suck in my gut and button them anyway, I think about my body *all day long.* (Because jeans that are too tight *hurt.* I can't breathe right and I get those horrible crease lines in my belly skin.) But when my jeans *fit,* I forget about my waistline and my mind is free to solve the problems of the world (or at least the problems of whatever script I'm working on). And the way you get your jeans to fit? Two choices: Buy bigger jeans (which I did for years until I was just south of clinically obese) or think for a few minutes at mealtime. That is seriously the trade-off. An all-day obsession vs. a few minutes each time you eat.

*Between half-listening to me talking to my teammate about carbohy-*
*drates and calories and "What a nice carbohydrate grapes are," and*

*half in his world of turbocharged-autobot-robotrons, my five-year-old
son announced, "Grapes are a great turbohydrate, Mom."*

—Jesse, 36

Okay, enough preamble. Here's what and how you're gonna be eating for the next four weeks, plain and simple.

# Your Meal Plan

Five meals a day, spaced out by anywhere from two to four hours. (Go more than four hours and you lose points!)

Each meal will consist of one lean protein, one healthy carb (like whole grains and fruits), one healthy fat, and as many green veggies as you want. But you must have at least two portions of veggies a day. (See the F.Y.T. food list in this chapter.)

The key to losing and not gaining weight when you're adding two extra meals a day is portion control. We have a HUGE (pun intended) problem with portion control in this country. We have supersized ourselves into a nationwide diabetic coma. Thank God Game On! is here to wake us all up!

## Determining Your Portion Size

Make a fist. Look at it. That's about how much carbs you should eat at each meal.

Now lay your hand flat and look at your palm (without your fingers and thumb). That's about how much protein you're gonna eat at each meal.

Now look at the size of your thumb. That's about how much healthy fat you'll add to each meal. (If you're eating oils, you'll eat only the amount of your thumb from the knuckle up! And keep in mind that butter and margarine are not healthy fats. See the food lists for your choices!)

If you are accustomed to eating the way most Americans have become accustomed to eating, these portions are going to feel very small to you in the beginning. But keep in mind—you get them five times a day. And—and this is a big *and*—you can eat as many green vegetables with each meal as you want! Eat a whole head of lettuce. Steam up four bags of spinach. I can't tell you how many times I've gotten tired of chewing and have still had veggies in my bowl. You will not go hungry, I promise.

Okay, ready? Here's the F.L.A.B.B. foods list. Remember—you get to indulge in these foods on your day off, your meal off, and your 100 calories a day of whatever. But it's important that you understand (as I was forced to, kicking and screaming) that you are *indulging* in them. They must become the exception to our dietary rules if we want a shot at long-term health and weight loss.

## F.L.A.B.B. (Fat-loading and Belly-bloating) Foods

All fried foods
High-fat/processed meats
Anything made with refined sugar (which includes sugar, corn syrup, high-
    fructose corn syrup, and sucrose)
Anything made with white flour
Butter
Margarine
Whole-fat cheese
Cream
Dried fruit/fruit juice **

### *Some common foods that fall into these categories:*
Baked goods
All sugary breakfast cereals
Most breakfast bars
Cakes
Candy
Chocolate
Condiments (ketchup, BBQ sauce, etc.)
Cookies
Donuts

Ice cream

Pastries

Pies

Granola**

Potato chips

French fries

Fruit "drinks"

Sugar-sweetened beverages

All sodas (Coke, Pepsi, etc.)*

All diet sodas*

Bacon

Fast-food sandwiches and burgers

Hot dogs

Jerky

Salami

Sausage

Bologna

Chicken nuggets, strips, fingers

Fish sticks

Mayonnaise

* not options for your 100 calories a day
** not junk food but *very* high calorie

As a general rule, the more processed and packaged and preserved it is, the worse it is for you. And the further away from *actual food* it is, the worse it is for you. We have not outlawed all artificial sweeteners, though we were veeeery tempted to. Instead, we are opting to give you all the information we can, and let you make the choice for yourself.

• • • • • • • • • • • • • • • • • • • • • • • • • • • • • • • • • • • • • •

## A word from Dr. David Katz

*I know there are factions out there who think artificial sweeteners are out-and-out poisons; I've heard from them each time I've addressed the topic publicly, such as on* Good Morning America. *My view is that the evidence for this is far from conclusive. However, I advise against artificial sweeteners because they are intensely sweet: 300 to 1,300 times as sweet as sugar! And we talk about a "sweet tooth," rather than a "sugar tooth," for good reason: It is sweet we crave. The more we get, the more we need—with pretty convincing evidence that sweet food is addictive, or nearly so. The result is that while artificial sweeteners take sugar and calories out of a food or drink, they don't reliably take them out of your diet! Your sweet tooth, grown into a sweet fang, will cause you to prefer sweeter foods and drinks in general, and those calories will sneak back in through side doors. There isn't consistent evidence that diet sodas or other artificially sweetened foods help with weight control. Animal research suggests they may actually do harm, which is also my impression based on years of experience with my patients. My advice to limit sugar is to look out for it in places it doesn't belong—such as pasta sauces, salad dressings, and even chips. Cut out superfluous sugar, and file a sweet tooth down to size.*

*—David L. Katz, MD, MPH, FACPM, FACP*
*Director, Prevention Research Center Yale University School of Medicine*

• • • • • • • • • • • • • • • • • • • • • • • • • • • • • • • • •

## F.Y.T. (Flatten Your Tummy) Foods

Are you screaming at me now? Are you all, NO SUGAR??? NO WHITE FLOUR?????? And you don't even want me to eat "diet" anything? SO WHAT THE HELL CAN I EAT, YOU CRAZY BITCH??? Sheesh . . . chilll . . . Here's a massive list of things you can eat! F.Y.T. foods are pronounced as "Fit," and they will keep you that way.

# The **GAME ON!** F.Y.T. Foods (Flatten Your Tummy Foods)

## Carbs!

Amaranth
Barley
Beans:
  Adzuki
  Black
  Black-eyed
  Broad
  Butter
  Fava
  Garbanzo (Chick Peas)
  Kidney
  Lentils
  Lima
  Mung
  Navy
  Pinto
  Soy
  White
Bran (Whole Grain)
Bread (Whole Grain)
Buckwheat (Whole Grain)
Bulgar (Whole Grain)
Corn
Crackers (Whole Grain)
Leek
Milk
Milk - Soy
Millet (Whole Grain)
Oatmeal (Whole Grain)
Palm Hearts
Parsnips
Pasta (Whole Grain)
Peas
Potato (Baked)
Potato (Sweet)
Pumpkin
Quinoa (Whole Grain)
Rice (Brown)
Rice (Wild)
Rye (Whole Grain)
Taro
Tortilla (Whole Grain)
Yams
Yoghurt (Fat-Free)

## Proteins!

**Dairy**
(Low Fat or Fat Free)
Cheese:
  American
  Cheddar
  Cottage
  Cream Cheese
  Feta
  Mozzarella
  Quark
  Ricotta
  Swiss

Egg Whites
Greek Yogurt

**Fish**
Anchovie
Catfish
Cod
Flounder
Hake
Halibut
Mackerel
Mahi Mahi
Perch
Salmon
Sardine
Snapper
Sole
Swordfish
Tilapia
Trout
Tuna

**Meat** (Lean Only)
Beef, Ground
Buffalo
Chicken Breast
Duck
Kangaroo
Lamb
Pork Tenderloin
Steak - Eye of Round

Steak - Flank
Steak - Top Round
Steak - Top Sirloin
Turkey Bacon
Turkey Breast
Turkey, Ground
Venison
Wild Game Meat

**Seafood**
Crab
Lobster
Mussels
Octopus
Oysters
Scallops
Shrimp
Squid

**Vegetarian** (Low Fat)
Seitan
Soy Foods
Tempeh
Tofu
Veggie Burgers

## Fats!

Avocado
Egg Yolk (one)
Olives
Nut Butters:
  Almond Butter
  Cashew Butter
  Peanut Butter
  Sesame Butter
  Sunflower Butter
Nuts (Dried/Raw):
  Acorns
  Almonds
  Beechnuts
  Brazilnuts
  Butternuts
  Cashews
  Hazelnuts
  Hickorynuts
  Macadamias
  Peanuts
  Pecans
  Pine Nuts
  Pistachio Nuts
  Walnuts
Seeds (Dried):
  Flax
  Pumpkin/Squash
  Safflower
  Sesame
  Sunflower
Oils:
  Fish Oils
  Flaxseed Oil
  Nut Oils
  Oil Spray (Pam)
  Olive Oils
  Udo's Oil
  Vegetable Oils

| CARBOHYDRATES: | PROTEIN: | FATS: |
|---|---|---|
| Eat a fist sized portion from the carbs or fruits list with every meal. | Eat a palm sized portion with every meal. | Eat a thumb-sized portion with every meal. |

# The **GAME ON!** F.Y.T. Foods (Flatten Your Tummy Foods)

## Veggies!

Alfalfa*
Artichoke
Asparagus*
Bamboo Shoot
Beans (Green)*
Beetroot
Broccoli*
Brussel Sprouts*
Cabbage*
Carrot
Cauliflower
Celery*
Chard (Swiss)*
Chinese Cabbage
Collards*
Cress
Cucumber*
Eggplant
Endive*
Fennel*
Gourd
Kale*
Lettuce*
Mushroom
Okra*
Onion
Peas (Snow)
Peppers
Pumpkin
Radish
Seaweed (Kelp)*
Spinach*
Squash(Summer)
Squash (Winter)
Tomatillo
Turnip
Watercress*
Zucchini*

## Fruits!

Apple
Apricot
Banana
Blackberry
Blueberry
Boysenberry
Cherimoya
Cherry
Clementine
Cranberry
Currant
Date
Durian
Fig
Gooseberry
Grape
Grapefruit
Guava
Huckleberry
Jack Fruit
Kiwi fruit
Kumquat
Lemon
Lime
Loquat
Lychee
Mandarin
Mango
Melon
Mulberry
Nectarine
Orange
Papaya
Passion Fruit
Peach
Pear
Persimmon
Pineapple
Plantain
Plum
Pomegranate
Quince
Rambutan

Raspberry
Rhubarb
Starfruit
Strawberry
Tamarillo
Tangerine
Tomato
Watermelon

## Sweeteners!

Agave Nectar
Honey
Pure Maple Syrup

**VEGETABLES:**
Add at least two fist-sized portions to at least two meals each day. You may eat unlimited greens (asterisked) with all of your meals.

**FRUITS:**
Eat a fist size portion from the carbs or fruits list with every meal.

**SWEETENERS:**
Use sweeteners very sparingly!

Use sweeteners very sparingly! Sweeteners are carbs and must be treated as such. If you are sweetening a meal, you must eat less of the carb to account for the amount of sweetener. Occasionally using a small drizzle is okay, but it's better to train your tastebuds to appreciate the natural sweetness in foods. The way you train your tastebuds is to cut out all sweeteners for a week or two. To understand just how caloric sweeteners can be, check out this ratio:

1 tablespoon of honey or agave nectar = about ⅔ of a medium-size potato.

1 tablespoon of maple syrup = just over ½ of a medium-size potato.

Sugar is a F.L.A.B.B. food because, as opposed to maple syrup, agave nectar, or honey, it has been stripped of all nutritional value. Artificial sweeteners are *strongly discouraged* as they are made of chemicals—and we proudly discourage the indiscriminate ingesting of chemicals. 'Cause, like, *ew*, y'know?

You are simply going to choose from the protein list, choose from the carbs or fruits list, and choose from the fats list—five times a day. To those meals, you can add as many veggies as you want—but *only* veggies from the veggies list! Potatoes may officially be a vegetable, but they're way too high calorie to eat in unlimited quantities.

It's simple, right? But here's the thing: The key to all of it is being aware of what's in the foods you're eating—and what I mean by that is, *you must know how they were prepared!* You would be amazed at how much diet-defeating crap can be hidden in what appears to be a healthy food. Like, if you go to a restaurant and order the sautéed spinach—the spinach itself has negligible calories. But the oil it's sautéed in? Adds hundreds and hundreds of calories to your dish. ORDER IT STEAMED. (And squeeze a little lemon juice on it to enhance the flavor.)

• • • • • • • • • • • • • • • • • • • • • • • • • • • • • • • • • • • • • • • • • • •

# High-Protein Vegan Foods

If you are a vegan, use these foods as your protein portion. Even though many of these are more carb than protein, they are all much higher in protein than your average carb. Please do NOT use nuts as your protein! They are far too high calorie to eat a palm-size portion. Eat nuts in small quantities (thumb-size) as your healthy fats.

| | | |
|---|---|---|
| Tempeh | Seitan | Soybeans |
| Lentils | Black beans | Kidney beans |
| Veggie burger | Chickpeas | Pinto beans |
| Black-eyed peas | Tofu | Lima beans |
| Quinoa | | |

• • • • • • • • • • • • • • • • • • • • • • • • • • • • • • • • • • • • •

## Diet Defeaters

Here for your horror (er . . . I mean, edification) is a list of really common sources of hidden calories.

### Soups

Broth soups are great (unless you see a bunch of oil floating in them), but if it looks creamy—run away!

### Coffee drinks

Black coffee is virtually calorie-free, but some coffee drinks can have as much as 1,000 calories in 16 ounces.

### Salad dressing

One tablespoon can have 50 to 80 calories and most of us are in the habit of using way more than one tablespoon. Also, many dressings have added sugar. Read the labels and use *sparingly.*

## Granola

Believe it or not, granola is often a fried food! The oats and nuts and dried fruits are sautéed in heavy oils—that's what makes them so rich. But a quarter-cup of granola often has several hundred calories—and we usually eat way more than a quarter-cup. Look for granolas that are BAKED and have no added sugars or preservatives.

## Fruit juice

Juice is high-calorie and the calories are empty of a lot of the nutrients provided by the whole fruit. Instead of a glass of O.J., you are way better served by eating an orange with your breakfast.

## Nuts

Nuts are excellent in many ways—but we tend to eat them by the handfuls. About 5 to 10 nuts is the most you want to eat with any meal. And even then, eat only raw or dry-roasted nuts to avoid added oils and sugar.

## Peanut butter

Just like nuts, all-natural (no sugar added) peanut butter can be a healthy and delicious treat—but it's a fat not a protein! A thumb-size portion is all your waistline can afford!

## Oils

They are used and overused in the preparation of so many foods, and they are incredibly high calorie. Read ingredients and, whenever possible, prepare your foods at home!

## Popcorn

Air-popped corn can be a delicious low-calorie carb. But prepared any other way, popcorn is loaded with high-calorie oils and usually loaded with various other flavoring chemicals like MSG. Save popcorn for the movies on your day off!

### Condiments

Condiments we use every day, like ketchup and barbeque sauce, add a staggering amount of calories to an otherwise healthy meal. Read the ingredients and when in doubt, avoid the sauce.

### Tuna salad

Tuna salad is a great source of protein—but the amount of mayo you'll find when you buy it on the road is diet-defeating. Make it at home and substitute a teaspoon of olive oil for mayo. Add a little salt and maybe some chopped celery or pickle and you'll have a delicious and healthy meal.

### Salads

Salads with cheese, bacon bits, and high-calorie dressings are NOT health foods. Which is why cheese, bacon bits, and high-cal dressings are not sanctioned foods!

### Dates and other dried fruits

They are so nutrient-rich but surprisingly high calorie. They are a great day-off treat! Also, read the ingredients—you want to make sure they don't have any added sugars. They're plenty sweet without them.

### Reduced-fat peanut butter

It has a lot of sugar and fillers and gross non-food food. It's a F.L.A.B.B. food for this reason.

### Whole-grain cereals

They can be healthy, but most people eat way more that one serving. Be SURE to stick to the portion rule here—no more than a fist-size amount.

### Margarine and butter

Both are startlingly high calorie. Save these foods for your day off.

### Smoothies

Do not order a smoothie without knowing what's in it! A little nonfat yogurt, whole fruit, and ice is a great thing. (And sometimes you can get a smoothie like this at your local health food store.) But many companies add ingredients like peanut butter and chocolate milk and ice cream and would have you believe it's a low-cal healthy snack. It's not. It's a dessert in a liquid form. These should be saved for your day off.

### Prep Time

So how do we do this? How do we avoid F.L.A.B.B. foods and hidden calories? Well, if you don't want to be the person in the restaurant ordering like this: *I'd like the asparagus and cheese omelet, but made with egg whites, and cooked in no butter, no oil, a little bit of cooking spray is okay. And no cheese please. Just the asparagus. And no potatoes on the side. I'd like fruit instead please. And no bread. Thank you!* then you should seriously consider preparing the bulk of your meals at home for the next four weeks. This may sound like a tall order, and again, it's not required, but it really does make the whole thing easier and save you from sounding like a neurotically skinny L.A. actress. (By the way, I am now the person in the restaurant ordering that way. Because despite preparing the best I can, my life still requires that I eat in restaurants sometimes. So I am super polite to the servers and I tip really, really well. Which is (a) the right thing to do and (b) the best way I know to avoid getting anyone's saliva in my food.)

• • • • • • • • • • • • • • • • • • • • • • • • • • • • • • • • • • • • • • • • • • •

## Tips for the Healthiest Preparation of Your F.Y.T. Foods

Bake or grill your protein.

Steam or bake your carbs and veggies.

Whenever possible, eat your fruits and veggies whole and raw. (Most of the nutrients are in the skin, and a lot of the nutrients get leached out in the cooking.)

Whenever possible, avoid heating your oils. High temperatures can change the molecular structure of the oil and change it from healthy to not so healthy. Consider baking or steaming your carbs and veggies and then drizzling room-temperature olive oil over the top.

• • • • • • • • • • • • • • • • • • • • • • • • • • • • • • • • • • • • • • • • • • •

So how do you prepare? Cook on Sunday night. Cook your meals for the whole week! Grill up a mess of chicken and a mess of fish and steam up a ton of veggies, slice up a bunch of fruit and a bunch of low-fat cheese and a whole bunch of celery and cucumber and make a big ol' vat of brown rice or quinoa or some other healthy grain. And then just grab a few Tupperwares every morning and pack up your meals for the day. If you are in the habit of getting take-out, you will not only save yourself a slew of hidden calories, you will also be actively saving the planet. Seriously, think about how much cardboard and plastic and Styrofoam you throw away every day! By treating your body well, you are treating Mother Earth well. It's win-win! (And if you are more of an actual cook than I am, we've included F.Y.T. food recipes at the end of this chapter! Yum!)

*I called Az prior to my marathon flight-day to North Carolina on Tuesday. I inquired as to which airport refreshments might fit into the game. He replied, "And why would you not pack your own meals?". . . My mind started spooling out all the excuses: got my six-year-old with me, already carrying a Sherpa-size load of stuff, have to pack his snacks, 30-minute layover, bla bla—but hey, the reality was, I wanted an excuse to eat a cardboard hot dog and chips, ok??!! So on Monday night I packed up in one multi-compartment Tupper-thingy two sanctioned meals, brown rice, tortilla, steak, chicken, salad, veggies, a little hummous, and a wee bit of oil/vin dressing—also had some Greek yogurt and a bunch of strawberries. Didn't really know how I was going to get my exercise, but the thirty-minute layover turned into a 20-minute layover and I ended up running the length of two concourses with a big backpack and my thirty-seven-pound son in my arms to make it to our next flight. My heart was literally beating out of my chest when we got to the gate (rounded out the exercise with a little power yoga when I got to my mom's). So it can be done, I now know. PS: got the water in too— that's what made the bag so damn heavy!*

  *Game on!*

*—Jes*

**Step Up Your Game!**

If you lose points on something small (say, you misread the in-gredients and ate a F.L.A.B.B. food) don't use it as an excuse to lose big! It's so tempting to say, "Oh hell, I lost my meal points already, I may as well eat some french fries too." But don't do it. I can tell you from experience that it doesn't make you feel any better. So instead, remind yourself of your goals. You are playing this game for a rea-son: You want to lose weight this week. And adding untold calories to justify a point loss won't help you reach that goal. Take a breath, eat the points and the points only, and move on.

So let's address the eating rules now.

## The Snacking Rule

Why are you allowed to snack on celery and cucumbers and nothing else? Because in the beginning, before your body has adjusted to your new por-tion sizing, or perhaps because you are sizing your portions slightly too small, you may suffer hunger pangs between meals. And the goal of the game is *not* to distract you from your work or family life with lingering hun-ger pangs. Cucumbers and celery are both very low calorie, plus full of water and high in fiber. They will fill you up and sate your hunger while adding a lot of nutritive value and without adding much in the way of calories. Az is urging me to add here that eventually, you won't need these foods between your meals because you will get better at knowing what kind of portions you need to tide you over till your next meal. But *he* is not orally fixated. Those of you who are all about chewing on something may never give up the cel-ery. And to you, I say, better a celery stalk than a cigarette or a Twinkie!

# The 100 Calories of Whatever You Want Rule

You can read more about it in Chapter 15, but I'll say here that this rule is largely in place to prevent the feelings of deprivation that come along with many diets. I cannot count how many times in my life I've deprived myself on some diet or other and then gotten so fed up with the deprivation that I eat waaaay more dessert than I ever would have had I not been depriving myself to begin with. (Once, when I was in high school and working an after-school job at a small bakery, I ate an entire banana cream pie. Not all at once, mind you. Just small slice by small slice over the course of my four-hour shift. Whole pie. Try explaining that to your boss.)

Because you can't generally measure calories in a birthday cake or homemade ice cream, a good rule on this is the *rule of thumb*—eat no larger a portion than the size of your thumb and you should be within your 100-calorie limit on just about any dessert. It's just a taste. Relish it.

## • • • Az's Shopping List • • •

Choosing organic as often as possible is a great way to go. Start with organic meat, poultry, fish, and eggs from cage-free hens, and then buy fresh, locally grown, organic fruits and veggies. (To find a farmers' market near you, go to www.localharvest.org.)

### Vegetables (fresh or frozen):
3 cucumbers
3 bunches of celery
1 head of lettuce
1 pound of mushrooms
2 pounds of tomatoes
1 bag or bundle of carrots
2 bags or bundles of fresh spinach
1 bundle of asparagus

2 bundles or bags of broccoli
1 bag of green beans

**Fruits:**
Apples
Bananas
Grapefruit
Lemons
Oranges
Pears
Peaches
Plums
Strawberries
1 bag of frozen mixed berries

**Grains and other carbohydrates:**
1 package whole grain oatmeal (not instant, nothing added)
1 package whole grain tortillas *or*
1 loaf whole grain bread
1 package whole grain hamburger buns
1 bag brown rice (*not* instant)
Small bag of potatoes
Small bag of sweet potatoes
Whole-grain pasta
Canned beans

**Meats, seafood, and other proteins:**
Skinless chicken breasts
Tuna steak or canned tuna
Lean cut of topside sirloin
Eggs from cage-free hens
Tofu
Low-fat mozzarella sticks
Low-fat milk

Nonfat Greek yogurt
Low-fat cottage cheese

**Healthy fats:**
Avocados
Almonds
Cashews
Walnuts
1 bottle of flaxseed oil
1 cup of fresh olives (canned or jarred olives are okay too—but
try to find them without added chemical preservatives)
Olive oil cooking spray
All-natural peanut butter

**Backup:**
Find some organic protein/food bars with as few added chemicals, sweeteners, etc., as you can. They actually have some that are
natural with a nice balance of protein, carbs, and healthy fats—so
read the ingredients and look for them!

**Condiments, herbs, and spices:**
Basil
Dill
Garlic
Ginger
Honey (or maple syrup)
Mustard
Pepper
Salt

When you get home, put all of your fresh fruit and vegetables
in the sink and soak them in filtered water and fresh lemon juice for
20 minutes, then rinse them again in filtered water. Even organic
vegetables are covered in various pesticides and chemicals (but you
should still buy organic whenever possible!). As a sidenote, floating

the fruit from a fresh lemon in your drinking water is a lovely idea—but the rinds of these fruits are covered in pesticides, which you definitely don't want leaching out into your drinking water! If you want to float the rinds of any fruit in your drinking water, be sure to soak the whole fruits (oranges, lemons) in lemon juice and water for a full 20 minutes and then rinse thoroughly.

• • • • • • • • • • • • • • • • • • • • • • • • • • • • • • • • • • • • • • • • • •

## A word from weight-loss coach Jennifer Kelman

*All of us have been guilty at one time or another of mindless munching. When mindless munching takes over, we are no longer enjoying our food, we are just shoveling it in. Becoming aware of your eating and bringing it back to a place of enjoyment will help with any weight-loss goals. Awareness helps us to feel satisfied and eat less. I suggest slowing down and getting your senses involved in the eating process. When was the last time you really tasted what you were eating or fully chewed your food? Pay attention to how each bite tastes and savor each delicious morsel. Closing your eyes for a moment while chewing can help put this into practice. Slow down, taste, and savor each bite. You will begin to notice that your satisfaction increases, which will prevent overeating and help in your weight-loss efforts.*

*—Jennifer L. Kelman, LMSW,*
*a clinical social worker and weight-loss coach*

• • • • • • • • • • • • • • • • • • • • • • • • • • • • • • • •

## The Five Meals a Day Rule

Finally, why are we suggesting five meals instead of three? Because, as we've mentioned, weight loss comes down to one thing and one thing ONLY. We must burn more energy than we consume. And the key to burning energy *faster* is the metabolism. As I have come to understand it, the best way to speed up the metabolism—in addition to exercising more—is to keep it clicking on all cylinders. And the way to do that is to always give it just enough food. Giving it too much food at once slows it down. When you have a couple of huge meals, it's like driving your car through mud—it's weighted down. When you have several small meals, it's like driving your zippy hybrid vehicle along traffic-free freeways, ocean air pouring in your windows. Wow. Clearly, I am not a doctor (and not much of a writer today, apparently). So let's hear what someone who actually knows something has to say . . .

• • • • • • • • • • • • • • • • • • • • • • • • • • • • • • • • • • • • • • • • •

## A word from Dr. David Katz

*We burn calories in three ways: basal metabolism, which is the energy cost of being alive; physical activity; and the generation of heat, known technically as "postprandial thermogenesis." That "postprandial" part is important: It means after meals. So by eating small meals spaced evenly throughout the day, you can keep those home fires burning, and use them to burn up some extra calories. The generation of heat accounts for some 15 percent of the calories we expend each day.*

*Other strategies for increasing metabolism include resistance training, which builds muscle, and eating complex carbohydrates and lean proteins. For every pound of muscle you add to your body, you need an extra 30 to 50 calories a day to maintain your weight. That means, do some resistance training a few times a week and burn more calories even in your sleep! As for food choices, complex carbohydrates, such as whole grains, contain fiber, which increases the work of metabolism. Protein, too, requires extra metabolic effort. This means more calories in foods such as whole grains or vegetables or fish are burned up while eating them than is the case for processed foods, and fewer are available to go into fat reserves.*

*—David L. Katz, MD, MPH, FACPM, FACP*
*Director, Prevention Research Center Yale University School of Medicine*

• • • • • • • • • • • • • • • • • • • • • • • • • • • • • • • • • • • •

My final tip for you is this: Know yourself. Know your needs. Know your day. Your meals do not have to be of equal sizes! The fist-palm-thumb thing is a great guideline, but you can be creative. If you know you have to go out for a work dinner and might eat a little more, eat a little lighter at meals 2 and 3. You can even think of your five meals as three meals and two snacks. Az's final meal is usually very light—some string cheese, a plum, and a few nuts. My final meal is usually a little more dessert—a little bit of oatmeal cooked up with an egg white, a few nuts, and a dash of maple syrup and cinnamon. It's a balanced meal, and I keep it small, but it satisfies my urge for a little something sweet at night. In general, you might want to eat a little more for your early meals and a little less for your later meals. The less you eat later in the day, the better you will sleep and the better it will be for your metabolism. And listen, *you can do this.* I know it's a lot of information, and it may seem like a lot of change, but I promise you, it will only take a few days—then you'll have it down and you will feel better. And when you feel better, life feels better. Seriously. In the meantime, here are a few sample recipes from former players to get you started.

Note: These recipes are written by players whose hands are of all different sizes. You may need to adjust the portion size of various ingredients according to the size of your own hand.

## Breakfast (Meal #1)
• • • • • • • • • • • • •

### Peter's Perfect Oatmeal Puddin' Breakfast

*Makes 1 serving*

½ *cup oats (not instant)*
3 *egg whites*
½ *cup fruit (blueberries, strawberries, peaches, whatever you have, fresh or*
    *frozen)*
1 *teaspoon flaxseed oil*
*A couple drops stevia or 1 teaspoon maple syrup*

Cook the oatmeal. While it's still on the heat and almost ready for serving, stir in the egg whites. Continue cooking for a minute or so more to make sure the egg whites cook through. Turn off the heat and add the fruit, flax-seed oil, and stevia or maple syrup. Hearty, tasty breakfast goodness.

## Krista's Quick and Easy Breakfast

*Makes 1 serving*

*Olive oil cooking spray*
*A few big handfuls of spinach*
*1 finely chopped onion*
*2 egg whites*
*1 or 2 teaspoons crumbled low-fat feta cheese*
*Salt and pepper to taste*
*1 slice whole grain toast*
*1 teaspoon olive oil*

Lightly spray a nonstick pan with the olive oil cooking spray. Over medium heat, sauté the spinach and onion until the spinach is wilted down and the onion is cooked through. Add the egg whites to the pan. When the egg whites are cooked through, crumble in the low-fat feta cheese, and add the salt and pepper to taste. Serve with one slice whole grain toast drizzled with the olive oil and lightly salted. Yum!

## Jana's Hearty Breakfast

*Makes 1 serving*

*As many veggies as you're hungry for (cabbage, snow peas, bok choy, etc. Fresh or frozen)*
*1 teaspoon olive oil*
*3 egg whites*
*¼ cup cooked brown rice*
*Dash of Bragg Liquid Aminos or soy sauce*

Over medium heat, lightly sauté the veggies in the olive oil. When the veggies are fork tender, add the egg whites. Continue cooking until egg whites

have been cooked through, and add the brown rice. Top with the Bragg
Liquid Aminos or soy sauce. Enjoy!

## Snacks (Meal #2 and/or #4)
• • • • • • • • • • • • • • • • •

### Az's Easy No-Cook Meal

*Makes 1 serving*

*2 low-fat cheese sticks (string cheese)*
*6 to 8 raw cashews*
*An apple and a plum*
*Or*
*A banana*

### Bill's Spicy Stuffed Pepper to Go

*Makes 1 serving*

When what you want is protein and vegetables, but you're running out the
door, you need something with the portability of, like, an apple. This recipe
provides you with that portability but way more protein!

*1 bell pepper (preferably yellow, red, or orange)*
*1 teaspoon Dijon mustard or garlic aioli*
*2 slices turkey breast*
*1 teaspoon olive oil or four olives*
*1 cup low-fat milk*

Pop out the stem and shake out the seeds of the pepper. Spread the Dijon
mustard or garlic aioli on the slices of turkey. Roll the turkey slices and stuff
them into the pepper. Drizzle the olive oil or stuff the olives into the pepper
for your healthy fat. Drink your glass of milk then scarf the rest on the run.
Crisp, refreshing, filling, delicious, fast food.

# Big Fella Phil's Banana Chocolate Protein Bars

*Makes 8 servings*

*Olive oil cooking spray*
*1 cup oatmeal*
*5 scoops (1 ounce each) chocolate protein powder*
*½ cup nonfat dry milk powder*
*2 egg whites*
*¼ cup fat-free cottage cheese*
*2 bananas, mashed*
*4 tablespoons water*
*2 tablespoons Agave Nectar*
*1½ teaspoon Udo's oil*
*Dash of vanilla extract*
*¼ cup raw, crushed almonds*

Preheat oven to 325°F and spray a 9 x 12 inch casserole dish with the cooking spray.

In a medium bowl combine the oatmeal, chocolate protein powder, and milk powder. In a separate mixing bowl beat the egg whites, then add the cottage cheese, bananas, water, Agave Nectar, oil, and vanilla extract until blended. Fold the dry ingredients into the wet ingredients and mix to combine. Pour the mixture into the pan, sprinkle the almonds on top, and bake for 30 minutes or until edges are browned. To serve, cut into 2 x 3 inch bars.

# Az's Super-Smooth Smoothie

*Makes 1 serving*

*1 cup either fat-free milk or soy milk*
*1 banana peeled and frozen or any other fruit (frozen strawberries are awesome too!)*
*6 almonds or 1 teaspoon flaxseed oil*
*½ cup fat-free Greek yogurt*
*1 pinch cinnamon*

Combine all ingredients in your blender and puree until smooth. Try it! It's a whole meal and it's delicious!

# Lunch (Meal #3)
· · · · · · · · · · ·

## Aussie Jo's Surf 'n' Turf salad
*Makes 1 serving*

Mix the following ingredients in the biggest salad bowl you have and toss with the delicious dressing.

### Salad

*½ head of romaine lettuce (the greener end, give the other end to your house mate, heheh)*
*1 green onion, chopped*
*1 tomato (nice and red for full flavor)*
*3 or 4 peperoncini*
*Cucumber slices, to taste*
*1 stalk celery, chopped*
*1 small carrot, chopped*
*¼ can unsweetened corn*
*3 artichoke hearts (we suggest you use the canned version)*
*½ a palm-size portion of chicken*
*½ a palm-size portion of tuna*

### Dressing
*Makes 1 serving*

Whisk the following ingredients in a small mixing bowl. Be sure to mix the garlic and balsamic vinegar together first so the vinegar has time to work its magic on the garlic.

1 garlic clove, crushed
$^1/_8$ cup balsamic vinegar
Dash of soy sauce
1 teaspoon flaxseed or olive oil
Salt and pepper, to taste

## Richard's Popeye Salad

*Makes 4 servings*

12 ounce bag spinach
3 cans tuna (6 ounces each and packed in water, not oil)
1 can bean medley
14 crushed almonds OR 2 tablespoons roasted flaxseeds
Crushed red pepper or hot sauce to taste, if desired

Mix all ingredients in a big-ass bowl. Divide the salad into 4 containers. You've got 4 good, hearty spinach salad meals in no time flat.

## Billy's Spicy Tuna Salad

*Makes 1 serving*

1 can tuna (6 ounces, packed in water)
1 red bell pepper, chopped
$^1/_2$ onion, chopped
1 clove garlic, crushed
2 tablespoons Dijon mustard or spicy mustard
1 teaspoon lemon juice
1 pinch dill (essential!)
$^1/_4$ cup beans your choice, canned
1 teaspoon olive oil

Combine all ingredients in a mixing bowl. Serve on a bed of chopped lettuce of your choice.

## Kristen's Light and Yummy Vegetarian Salad
*Makes 1 serving*

*1 cup nonfat Greek yogurt*
*1 small (fist-size) boiled potato*
*1 whole cucumber*
*3 stalks celery*
*4 pitted olives, chopped*
*Chopped dill, to taste*
*Lemon juice, to taste*
*1 pinch salt*

Combine all ingredients in a mixing bowl. Experiment with the dill and lemon juice to change the flavor of this delish dish.

# Dinner (Meal #4)
• • • • • • • • • •

## Auntie Jo's Sneaky Soup
*Makes 1 serving*

*1 chicken or vegetable bouillon cube*
*1 green onion, finely chopped*
*1 celery stalk, finely chopped*

In a deep pan on medium heat, dissolve the bouillon in 1 cup of hot water. Stir in the finely chopped green onion and celery and simmer for a few minutes. Drink with any meal to feel like you've had a soup starter! (The whole cup will have fewer than ten calories!)

## Jesse's Famous Turkey and Veggie Burgers
*Makes 4 to 6 servings, depending on the size of your palm*

*Virgin coconut oil (to brush onto parchment paper)*
*1 pound lean ground turkey*

*1 small maui sweet onion, chopped*

*½ cup chopped red, yellow, or green peppers*

*1 cup chopped spinach*

*1 tablespoon egg whites*

*⅛ teaspoon sea salt*

*⅛ teaspoon white pepper*

*1 pinch dried oregano, dried thyme, or a spice mélange such as 21 Salute from Trader Joe's, or Spike (avoid spice mixes with high sodium . . . and run from MSG)*

*Several 1-inch pieces of low fat-string cheese or low-fat feta cheese*

Preheat oven to 350°F and line a large glass casserole dish with parchment paper, brushed with a small amount (just dip a basting brush once) of virgin coconut oil.

In a medium mixing bowl combine all ingredients and mix by hand. Form patties that are the size and thickness of your palm. If you eat dairy, add a 1-inch piece of low-fat string cheese or low-fat feta cheese and push it into the center of the patty.

Bake patties for 20 to 25 minutes, or until the turkey turns white and is firm to the touch. Once cooked, transfer the patties to the broiler to brown the tops, and crisp any of the exposed veggies.

Serve sliced over chopped veggie salad or roasted green veggies. Add a fist-size portion of carbohydrate, such as roasted white or sweet potatoes on the side!

## Jesse's Game On! Chicken Lettuce Cups

*Makes 4 to 5 servings, depending on the size of your palm*

*2 cloves garlic, minced*

*2 tablespoons minced fresh ginger*

*2 tablespoons vegetable stock*

*3 to 4 tablespoons soy sauce*

*1½ tablespoons rice vinegar*

*1 teaspoon honey*

1 package ground white meat chicken
*⅓ cup chopped scallions*
*1½ yellow bell peppers, chopped*
*¼ cup chopped cilantro*
*2 or 3 drops sesame oil*
*¼ teaspoon red chili flakes, optional*
*One head of Bibb or romaine lettuce*
*Garnishes: Sesame seeds, crushed cashews, chopped cilantros, chopped scallion*

Sauté the garlic and ginger in vegetable stock over medium heat until soft, add more stock if pan gets too dry. In a small bowl, whisk the soy sauce, vinegar, and honey and set aside.

Add the chicken to the garlic and ginger and raise the cooking temperature to medium/high. Break the ground chicken into small crumbles with a spoon as it cooks. When the chicken changes color from pink to white add the soy mixture, scallions, and yellow peppers.

Cook the chicken mixture for approximately 5 more minutes. After 5 minutes, turn off the heat and add the cilantro, sesame oil, and optional chili flakes

While the mixture cools, wash and separate the lettuce leaves. Choose leaves that can accommodate ⅓ of a cup of the chicken mixture.

One Game On! Meal includes 2 lettuce cups, each filled with ⅓ cup of the chicken mixture. Garnish with a teaspoon of sesame seeds or 2 teaspoons of crushed cashews, chopped cilantro, and chopped scallion.

Serve with chopped veggie salad or roasted green veggies. Add a fist-size portion of carbohydrate, such as roasted white or sweet potato mixed in on the side.

Store extra prepped lettuce leaves in a plastic bag, wrapped in a moistened paper towel.

## Jesse's 'Mazing Marinade

This marinade can be used for pork, fish, shrimp, or steak and is good for broiling or grilling.

In a large Ziploc baggie mix:

*¼ cup soy sauce*
*1 tablespoon rice vinegar*
*3 tablespoons orange juice*
*⅛ teaspoon Chinese five-spice powder*
*¼ cup chopped scallions*
*2 cloves garlic, minced*
*2 tablespoons minced ginger*

Place your meat of choice (up to 2 pounds) into bag with marinade and let sit in the refrigerator for a minimum of 2 hours but preferably overnight.

## Mandy's Friggin' Awesome Chicken Cacciatore
*Makes 2 to 3 servings, depending on the size of your palm*

*1 spritz olive oil cooking spray*
*2 chicken breasts, chopped*
*1 onion, chopped*
*Italian seasoning, to taste*
*Salt and pepper, to taste*
*1 clove garlic, chopped*
*¼ cup white cooking wine*
*1 large can stewed tomatoes*
*1 can water (you can use the stewed tomatoes can to measure your water)*
*3 cups veggies (peas, carrots, broccoli, etc. Frozen is fine, but fresh is better)*

Spritz a medium-size pot with the olive oil spray, and brown the chicken over medium heat for just a few minutes (don't cook it through). Remove the chicken from the pot (don't clean the pot) and set aside.

To the same pot, add the onion, seasoning, salt and pepper to taste, and garlic. Saute for 30 seconds and add the white cooking wine. Continue to sauté for about a minute and a half to allow for the alcohol to cook off. Add the tomatoes, water, veggies, and chicken, and bring to a boil. Reduce heat and simmer for 20 minutes before serving.

It's healthy and great served over a little bit of brown rice!

## Brad's Most Excellent Cashew Mango Chicken

*Makes 1 serving*

1 chicken breast
½ cup light chicken stock
6 crushed cashews
Pepper, red pepper flakes, and garlic powder, to taste
1 mango
1 medium-size onion
1 bunch cilantro
1 cucumber
1 squeeze lime juice

Preheat oven to 350°F.

Lightly soak the chicken breast in the light chicken broth. Next, roll the chicken in the crushed cashews, pepper, red pepper flakes, garlic powder, and any other spices you love. Bake for 35 minutes.

While baking, chop up the mango, onion, cilantro, and cucumber and add a squeeze of lime juice. Once the chicken is ready, spoon the mango salsa over the top of the chicken and serve over steamed spinach and a side of your favorite veggies.

## Kate's Simply Skinny Sausage Supper

*Makes 1 serving*

Olive oil cooking spray
1 chicken sausage, sliced
1 fist-size portion of cooked brown rice
Steamed broccoli (all you want)

*A few dashes Bragg Liquid Aminos (a low-sodium, soy, yeast, and gluten-free soy sauce alternative)*

Sauté it all together in a nonstick pan with a touch of cooking spray. Yum!

## Jo's Bell Pepper of the Ball

*Makes 1 serving*

*1 red or green bell pepper*
*1 palm-size portion of extra-lean turkey or ground beef*
*¼ cup chopped onion*
*1 carrot, chopped*
*1 clove garlic, chopped*
*1 small tomato, chopped*
*Salt, pepper, and spices, to taste*
*Fist-size portion of brown rice or cooked beans of choice*

Preheat the oven to 350°F.

Slice the "lid" off the red or green bell pepper and shake out the seeds.

In a medium bowl, mix the extra lean turkey or ground beef with the chopped onion, carrot, garlic, oil, tomato, salt, pepper, and spices to your fancy. Add half a fist-size portion of either cooked rice or beans and mix well.

Stuff the mixture into the bell pepper and bake in the oven for 45 minutes with the lid on the pepper. Then remove the lid and bake the pepper for another 15 minutes.

Enjoy this meal with steamed broccoli or spinach as a side dish.

## Katie's Lemon Chicken Feast

*Makes 1 serving*

*¼ cup lemon juice*
*3 teaspoons Dijon mustard*
*1 chicken breast, cut into 4 or 5 thin slices*

In a small bowl, mix the lemon juice with the Dijon mustard.

In a nonstick pan, sauté the chicken in the lemon and mustard mixture until the chicken is cooked through.

Serve with a small sweet potato (baked or boiled) and a big green salad (for salad dressing, mix lemon juice with ¼ of a small avocado and stir it up until the avocado is liquid. Add salt, pepper, basil, and garlic powder to taste).

# Dessert (Meal #5)

## Brooke's Crunchfest 2009

*Makes 1 serving*

½ *cup plain yogurt*
½ *cup cottage cheese*
*Dash vanilla extract*
¼ *cup any kind of berry*
¼ *cup Kashi GoLean Crunch with Almonds*

In a bowl, combine the yogurt, cottage cheese, and vanilla extract. Top with the berries and Kashi GoLean Crunch.

## Kevin's Vanilla Strawberry Almost Ice Cream Treat

*Makes 1 serving*

½ *cup low-fat ricotta cheese*
½ *cup frozen strawberries (half-thawed)*
*Dash vanilla extract*
*2 teaspoons maple syrup*
*2 teaspoons crushed cashews or macadamia nuts*

Mix it all together and call it a day!

# Bill and Jana's Tropical Treat

*Makes 1 serving*

1 cup 0 percent Greek yogurt
½ cup frozen pineapple chunks
2 teaspoons shredded coconut

Mix and enjoy!

# Hammer's Blue Lagoon

*Makes 1 serving*

1 cup 0 percent Greek yogurt
½ cup fresh or frozen blueberries
2 teaspoons crushed walnuts

Tangy and delicious!

# Mandy's Party Time Popsicles—you heard me—POPSICLES!

*Makes 1 serving*

½ cup cottage cheese
½ cup 0 percent Greek yogurt
1 piece chopped fruit or 2 teaspoons honey (or half a piece of fruit and one
    teaspoon honey)
6 cashews

Blend it all together within an inch of its life. Freeze in Popsicle molds
and eat!

Note: The reason we have specified using 0 percent Greek yogurt in
certain recipes is because it is much higher in protein than regular yogurt. Therefore it qualifies as protein whereas other yogurts are counted
as carbs.

# Frequently Asked Questions

Q: If you eat F.L.A.B.B. food during a meal do you just lose the points for the meal or do you take a snacking penalty?

A: If you skip a meal, or eat F.L.A.B.B. foods during a meal, you just lose the six meal points. You take a snacking penalty only if you eat *between* meals.

Q: Can I play the game and do my Jenny Craig/Weight Watchers/South Beach Diet diet plan instead of the game diet plan?

A: Absolutely. Obviously, we like our meal plan best, but we're not snobs. If you want to apply our rules to your favorite diet/meal plan, be our guest. Just let your teammates and opponents know that that's how you intend to play. AND make sure you eat five times a day. That piece is really important.

Q. I'm a vegetarian and I hate eating protein at every meal because I end up eating too much soy. Can I still play?

A: Yes! BUT if you aren't eating protein at every meal, then you RE-ALLY need to count calories—because it's the lean proteins that really help keep the meals at a reasonable calorie count. Go to www.thegameondiet.com for help in counting calories. And simply inform your teammates that you will be playing by slightly modified rules.

Q: Why are fruit juice and dried fruits F.L.A.B.B. foods? Aren't they good for me?

A: The answer is Yes and No. Dried fruits are nutritionally sound (though inferior to fresh fruits) but they are very calorie dense. If you compare an equal amount of apples and dates—you get about five and a half times the number of calories in the dates. Because they are so high in natural sugars and so high in calories, dried fruits can be really diet defeating, which is why they're F.L.A.B.B. foods. As to fruit juice, what's happened there is that most of the fruit's nutrients and all of the fiber have been left in the flesh of the fruit and all you're getting is the sweet, high-calorie, natural liquid sugar. A glass of orange juice is about five oranges worth of juice—and is less satisfying and far less nutritional than just eating one whole orange. Stick with the whole fruit and your waistline will thank you!

Q: Why is white flour a F.L.A.B.B. food?

A: Refined white flour is basically wheat with everything healthy about it stripped away. It not only lacks nutrients, but the refinement process removes all fiber from the grain, which prompts white flour to behave like pure sugar when it enters the body. It's metabolized too quickly, causing blood glucose disturbances and sugar cravings. Eat too many of these foods and you will undoubtedly have mood swings and may get depressed, angry, and irritable. It's not good for your health, not good for your weight loss, not good. Stick to whole grains, whole wheat, or wheat alternatives like spelt.

Q: Why is sugar a F.L.A.B.B. food?

A: Like white flour, refined sugar is without nutritional value. In addition to adding untold empty calories to your diet, it rushes into your bloodstream and wreaks havoc with your blood sugar levels and makes losing weight much harder than it needs to be. It also causes mood swings and has been connected with many diseases—from Alzheimer's to cancer. Whenever possible, Just Say No.

Q: Why can't I have diet soda?? It's calorie-free!

A: Because we are trying to break you of the habit of drinking any soda at all. It's either full of sugar or full of chemicals or full of both. Calorie-free or not, it messes with your body's ability to function at maximum capacity.

Q: Give up diet soda?! Are you crazy? I can cut down, but I need the caffeine to get through my day. Can I at least drink one and use it as my 100 calories of whatever?

A:  No. But you can have a little coffee or some green tea or black tea, iced or hot, for a little caffeine blast. For a touch of sweet, you can stir in a teaspoon of honey or maple syrup.

Q:  Is it okay to skip the fat in my meal? Won't that help me lose weight quicker?

A:  No!! Healthy fats are an absolutely essential nutrient for weight loss. A new study shows that dieters who decreased calories while concentrating on healthy fats and carbohydrates had higher metabolisms after ten weeks of dieting and reported less hunger than dieters taking in the same number of calories who ate only low-fat foods.

Q:  What's the best way to measure the amount of butter I use on my toast? My thumb nail?

A:  Trick question, right? You trickster, you! Butter is a F.L.A.B.B. food. Try drizzling your toast with a teaspoon of olive oil and sprinkling a little salt on top. YUM!

Q:  I'm a teacher and I'm finding it really hard to eat five meals a day. I can't really be eating while I'm teaching.

A:  Believe me, after a few days of eating this way, you'll be really hungry every few hours and eager to find ways to get your sustenance (even if it means giving your students a "pop quiz" so you can turn your back to them and eat your protein bar or drink your homemade smoothie while they cheat!).

Q:  Do I have to have a protein, carb, and fat in EVERY meal? Like, I can't just have salad?

A:  You can just have salad. Just throw some egg whites or tuna on top, sprinkle some chopped apples on it, and use a teaspoon of an olive oil–based dressing and you've got a perfect meal! There are so many salads you can make—and combining the foods is really easy after a few days. Do your best to follow the meal plan as closely as you can—because I'm telling you, it works!

## Play by the Rules

- Eat five small meals a day. Use your palm, fist, and thumb to determine portion size.
- Eat a lean protein, a healthy carb, and a healthy fat with each meal.
- Eat F.Y.T. foods. Don't eat F.L.A.B.B. foods.
- You may eat as many leafy green vegetables with each meal as you desire. This is in addition to your carb/fruit portion (not in place of it.)
- Read ingredients lists carefully.
- Eat "whole" foods—whole grains, fruits, vegetables—as much as possible.
- Eat organic foods as often as possible.
- Before eating, soak your fruits and veggies in lemon juice and water to eliminate pesticides and impurities.
- Between meals, you may snack on celery and cucumbers without penalty. Eating anything else between meals incurs a snacking penalty.
- If you find that you are frequently hungry, add more vegetables to your meals.
- The more time you put in planning ahead and preparing your meals, the easier your day will be.
- When dining out, be very aware of how the foods you're ordering are prepared—even if it means annoying the waiter.
- When you annoy the waiter, be as polite as possible and then tip well.

# Chapter 9

# EXERCISE

## (Or, I Never Even Knew I Had a Muscle There.)

I gotta work out. I keep saying it all the time.
I keep saying I gotta start working out.
It's been about two months since I've worked
out. And I just don't have the time. Which is
odd. Because I have the time to go out to
dinner. And watch TV. And get a bone
density test. And try to figure out what my
phone number spells in words.

—*Ellen DeGeneres*

> **The Rule:** You must exercise (any kind of exercise that makes your breathing speed up) for a minimum of 20 minutes a day, six days a week, to earn 20 points a day.
>
> You may do a seventh day of exercise but you will not earn extra points.

**Exercise. Not my** thing. Really, really, super not my thing. I ran track my freshman year of high school because my sister Kaili was a track star and I used to like to copy everything she did. (Also, there was a boy I liked on the track team. Chris McSomething. Tall. Irish. Cuuuute.) But when the coach would make us run two miles around the neighborhood every day after school as a "warm up," I would run the quarter-mile to the local Dunkin' Donuts, eat an Old-Fashioned Buttermilk Cruller, and hang out until I saw some kids heading back to school. Then I would fall in line with them and run the quarter-mile back, panting vigorously and often cramping from running with fresh donut in my stomach. True story. (Also, when we were kids Kaili was a gymnastics star so I followed her to gymnastics class. After four years of lessons I still couldn't do a cartwheel. And can't to this day.)

*After watching* The Secret *I was convinced I could increase my metabolism with mantras such as "Pizza digests perfectly and quickly in my body." Didn't work. Exercise works better. And the game made me willing to exercise.*

—Tammy, 39

Not much has changed since then. In my office today, I have a giant, squishy, green reclining chair with this fabulous fabric that, no matter what you spill on it, always stays clean. I love this chair. I live in this chair. One of the writers I work with recently suggested that I should have a picture of feet on my business card, because that's all he ever sees of me—my feet on the end of my reclining chair as he walks past my office. The nature of my job is that I often have to write twenty, thirty, even forty pages in a day, up against tight deadlines. What this means is that on a writing day, which is most days, I sit in my chair for somewhere between eight and twelve hours, only ever getting up to race to the bathroom and back. Every few hours, my assistant brings me food, which I eat with one hand while typing with the other.

There is no time, no option for any kind of exercise. Believe me, I'm not complaining, I'm just explaining. If exercise were my thing, I might complain. But as I mentioned above: really, really, super not my thing. I am truly happy in my fluffy green chair with the adrenaline of looming deadlines surging through my blood. If I could get away with never exercising and stay healthy and reasonably fit? I would not have a problem with that. Happy, happy, happy to sit still.

The thing is: I *can't* get away with never exercising and stay healthy and reasonably fit. I know this because, as I've mentioned, when I moved to Hollywood to be a TV writer, I weighed about 155 pounds, and by the time I got pregnant eight years later, I weighed 185 pounds—after losing five pounds at a juice spa.

*Nobody hated exercise more than I did, and when I read that I had to exercise for 20 minutes a day to win, I thought I'd just read that O.J. was coming over. But a girl's gotta do what a girl's gotta do, so I strapped on the running shoes and went, and it changed my life immensely! I didn't feel like I needed to sleep more when I woke up in the morning. I had incredible energy throughout the day. My once squishy tummy became more toned and the euphoric feeling I got after only 20 minutes of moving my body was enough to keep me exercising daily, even after the game ended!*

—Star, 22

Before I became a working writer I had time in my day and I would often go for a hike with a friend who was walking her dog, or to the gym because another friend was teaching a spinning class. I would also move around a lot just in daily activity—walking to a restaurant for lunch, playing Frisbee on the beach with my boyfriend, boogie boarding in the ocean with friends, or Rollerblading with my sister around Central Park. (I was also a waitress for years and I swear on any given shift you walk five miles between the kitchen and the bar and your tables.) Exercise wasn't my thing even then, but I naturally kept my weight in a healthy range because I was often in motion.

And then I got my first job in television.

The end.


By the time Az came into my life I had myself convinced that it was humanly impossible to do my job and get any kind of exercise ever. He said, What about working out in the morning before work? I said, That's time I could be with my daughter. He said, How about over your lunch hour? I said, I write through my lunch hour. He said, What about at night? I said, I'm tired at night. He said, Krista, I'm asking you for 20 minutes. Just 20 minutes of putting your body in motion. You can go for a fast walk after dinner. You can do sit-ups and push-ups on the floor beside your baby while she sleeps. You can jump around your living room or you can jump on to your dusty home-exercise equipment. Any time of day or night. For 20 minutes. *You really can't find 20 minutes?*

Even I couldn't pretend that I couldn't find 20 minutes. When I started to pay attention, I noticed that even on my busiest deadline days, I would stop writing to check e-mails or read *People* online. The human brain cannot focus on one thing for twelve hours in a row. You get about two hours before your brain starts to wander, your writing gets bad, and you need a reboot. My habitual reboot was e-mailing and checking up on celebrity gossip. Az was asking me to get up out of my fluffy green chair and exercise instead. Still, I'm a rebel and I resist change, so I didn't exercise every day until Az proposed the game. There are big points—20 POINTS A DAY—attached to those 20 minutes of exercise. A POINT PER MINUTE!

Exercise is not my thing. Winning is. So I started to move my body six days a week for 20 minutes each day. I hate exercising in the morning so I didn't often do it despite Az's insistence that it has more benefit. (It jump-starts your metabolism, prompting you to burn more calories throughout the day.) Most often, I would get my exercise at night. Az taught me a hard, 20-minute high-intensity interval training (HIIT) workout that I would do two or three days a week. (You'll see how to do it later in this chapter.) On the other days, I would dance around the house with my baby or do calisthenics on the floor of her nursery while she lobbed balls at my head, or, after she'd go to sleep, I would jump on the stationary bike. Some days I would take a fast walk around my neighborhood at lunch (because I dis-covered that I write more and better when there's a little extra blood flow-ing to my brain). Some days I would put on music and lock the door and jump around my office. (My current favorite workout song? "*Hey! Hey! You! You! I don't like your girlfriend . . .*" Avril Lavigne. I'm not proud.)

I should mention that there were and are very real added benefits to forcing myself to do the 20 minutes no matter how tired or cranky I am. One is that I'm always less tired and less cranky when I'm done. The other is that I actually sometimes don't stop at 20 minutes 'cause it feels so good to move. The third is that I'm way less fat.

Come on. Join me in Way Less Fat Land. It's nice here! And easier to breathe!

## • • • A Tip from Az • • •

When Krista and I had the conversation she's recounted, she was weighing 205 pounds—the "before" picture you've seen in this book. She was more than 50 pounds overweight.

At that weight, 20 minutes of any exercise can make a big dif-ference. At that weight, your body has to work so hard and burn so many calories just to carry the extra weight around that *when you combine exercise with a sensible diet* it's actually easier to lose weight.

If you are closer to your goal weight—within twenty pounds—you will have to do a more vigorous exercise routine if you want to meet your weekly weight-loss goal. Still, you can keep it to 20 minutes a day and see results! All the new research is saying that results are less about how *long* you exercise than how *hard* you exercise.

The very best aerobic workout you can get is 20 minutes of high-intensity interval training (HIIT). There are a bunch of ways to do it, and I've outlined several of them on the following pages.

• • • • • • • • • • • • • • • • • • • • • • • • • • • • • • • • • • • • • • • •

## A word from *Grey's Anatomy*'s own overachieving doctor/writer/producer, Dr. Zoanne Clack

*As an emergency medicine physician, I wish I could drill three things into the minds of every person everywhere:*

1. *Wear your damn seatbelt!*
2. *Don't abuse your children!*
3. *Exercise more!*

*I'm not sure that's the right order. I might do away with child abuse first—but you get the idea. And you'll notice that all three things on this list are DO-ABLE. You don't hear me yelling at you not to develop Parkinson's or not to get cystic fibrosis. I am yelling about things each and every one of us has the power to change. And if you're looking at number 2 and you're saying, "Well, no way in hell would I abuse my child," then look at number 3 and consider the fact that by eating crappy foods and refusing to move your body, you are abusing somebody's child: your parents' child. (God's child? Both?)*

*On any given night, the ER is filled with men and women coming in with the agony of a heart gone bad. Young men and young women. Men and women with children and spouses and parents who love them. Men and women who have NO BUSINESS having heart attacks, but here they are anyway, having heart attacks in my ER. Heart attacks, by the way, that likely would not have happened if the patient didn't have (a) high blood pressure, (b) high cholesterol, or (c) type II diabetes.*

*Exercise can help you prevent or manage or undo all of those abc's I listed. It also slows down aging, decreases your risk of Alzheimer's, reduces your need for prescription drugs, and can even help to make your heart and lungs stronger. Exercise will help you become more active, more energized, and more vital; you'll sleep better, you'll look better, you'll feel better. It is the ONE thing you can do to completely change your life and health!*

*And listen, I know I sound a little preachy, but I'm not talking to you as some skinny chick who's never had a weight issue of her own. I'm speaking to you as a woman who at the age of forty said Enough! and lost more than fifty pounds. And I'm speaking to you as a person who, when I hit a weight-loss plateau, played Krista and Az's game to push through it. I'm healthier and more fit at forty than I've ever been in my life. Why? Because (a) I wanted to look great (and now I do), (b) I was tired of hiding behind the fat and making excuses for why my clothes didn't fit and my social life was in the toilet, and (c) I didn't want to end up a heart attack in someone else's ER. (Again, not necessarily in that order.)*

*—Zoanne Clack, MD, MPH, FACEP*

• • • • • • • • • • • • • • • • • • • • • • • • • • • • • • • •

## Motivation

Okay, so hopefully the doctor has convinced you that you *should* be exercising. But knowing you should do it and *doing* it are two different things. For me, the added motivation, besides winning points and obliterating my opponents, is about music.

MUSIC is truly the difference for me between enjoying a workout and hating every minute of it. It is also the difference between working out at half speed (if the music is too slow) and full throttle (if the music is, say, REM's "It's the End of the World as We Know It"). Seriously, I can be on the stationary bike and think I am riding as hard and fast as I can. And then a much faster song starts to play, and suddenly I am riding much harder and much faster. So my suggestion is that you get a bunch of fast songs that you love. And in case you're not sure where to start, here's a little assist from my favorite spinning instructor.

• • • • • • • • • • • • • • • • • • • • • • • • • • • • • • • • • • • • • • • • • • • • • • •

# A word from spinning instructor Sue Molnar

*Since I believe that MUSIC can turn an average, arduous "workout" into a transformative, joyous experience, I think that if people can find music that is particularly inspiring to them (at home or in a group exercise format) they might just trick themselves into enjoying exercise after all.*

*Trying to force yourself to exercise or work out when you don't enjoy it is riding the horse backwards. It is self-defeating. Once you figure out a way to make exercise not only tolerable, but enjoyable and thrilling, which is what the right music does for me, you're finally riding the horse in the right direction. You're naturally transported to a place of better fitness, greater stress relief, more energy, a better sex life, a stronger heart, increased self-esteem, the ability to eat the foods you love without worrying about your waistline . . . the list goes on.*

*Of course, any list is going to be arguable, but I just went through my iPod, which is filled with music culled over my past fifteen years as a fitness instructor, and picked the songs that have consistently been received with the most enthusiasm over the years. Here they are—in no particular order.*

1. "Unleashed"—Chris Classic
2. "Lose Yourself"—Eminem
3. "No More Drama"—Mary J. Blige
4. "Bawitdaba"—Kid Rock
5. "Wanna Be Startin' Somethin'"—Michael Jackson
6. "Gonna Fly Now" (Theme from *Rocky*)—Bill Conti
7. "Stronger"—Kanye West
8. "Bodies"—Drowning Pool
9. "Freedom"—George Michael
10. "Hazy Shade of Winter"—The Bangles
11. "River Deep, Mountain High" (Live)—Celine Dion
12. "Proud Mary"—Ike & Tina Turner
13. "Good Vibrations"—Loleatta Holloway & Marky Mark & The Funky Bunch
14. "Gloria"—Laura Branigan

15. "Mamma Mia"—Abba
16. "Hush"—Kula Shaker
17. "I Just Want to Celebrate"—Rare Earth
18. "Heroes"—U-Traxx
19. "Hurricane 2000"—Scorpions & Berliner Philharmoniker
20. "Fame 02"—Tommy Lee

*Have a great workout, y'all!*

—*Sue Molnar, spinning instructor, Soul Cycle, New York City*
*For more music and fitness tips, go to www.SuesTrax.com*

• • • • • • • • • • • • • • • • • • • • • • • • • • • • • • • •

So it's music that motivates me. Figure out what motivates you. Here's a list of possibilities.

- Do you need new workout clothes 'cause you like the added possibility of meeting your soul mate at the gym? Buy them!
- Do you need a new gym membership 'cause all the guys at your gym are gay (and you're not)? Get one!
- Do you need new shoes so you can run faster/longer/better? Buy them today. It's an investment in your health.
- Do you require a workout buddy—someone to show up for or who will show up for you? Ask a teammate or opponent to be your person.
- Don't know what you and your workout buddy will talk about while you run around the park? Read the same book for your healthy habit—and then you can have a running book club.
- Do you love to read but don't have time? Download an audio book to your iPod. Make it a scary one, and you'll run even faster!
- Do you need a good excuse to read trashy celebrity gossip magazines? Give yourself permission to read them on the stationary bike—as long as you keep your effort at 80 percent or more.
- Do you have a friend you haven't seen in ages and feel like you have

no time to catch up? Ask her to meet you for a hike or a fast walk in the local park before or after work.

BE CREATIVE. Most of us don't exercise because we think it's boring and/or time we could be spending doing other things. So make it not boring—and combine it with other things! For me, it's both workout and mental health break. Getting my heart rate up while shouting Avril Lavigne lyrics makes me feel better in about sixteen different ways. Believe it or not, I look forward to it now. I actually *enjoy it*. Almost as much as I enjoy camping out in my squishy green chair.

### • • • A High-Intensity Interval Training • • • Session with Az!

Studies show that high-intensity interval training (HIIT) is by far the most efficient way to burn calories and maximize weight loss.

HIIT is so effective because it raises your heartbeat to close to your maximum, and in doing so, it raises your resting metabolic rate. That means you're *burning calories at a higher rate for up to twenty-four hours after your exercise*. And the best part is that you get this benefit in only a 20-minute workout! As with most things in life, your best workout is about quality not quantity.

So how do you do it? You simply vary your pace from minute to minute, or in ten- or twenty- or thirty-second segments. That's it! And you can apply this principle to any form of workout you can imagine.

If you're at the walking level, then you simply pick a landmark, like a telephone pole, and you walk as quickly as you can to that point. Then you pick another landmark and walk there at a moderate pace to recover. Then you pick another landmark and walk as quickly as you can again, and so on until your 20 minutes is up.

If you're riding a stationary bike or using a Stairmaster or running on a treadmill, alternate between riding/climbing/running at your hardest pace for 30 seconds, then drop back down to about 60 percent for 30 seconds, then back up again.

If you're swimming, swim as hard and fast as you can for a lap and then cruise for the next and so on.

If you're cycling, then cycle as quickly as you can for 30 seconds, and then cruise for 30 seconds to recover.

If you're pushing a stroller, push it as fast as you can for 30 seconds and then amble for 30 seconds to recover. (Your kids will love it and giggle all the way!)

Again, if you don't have a watch handy you can just pick landmarks. Go as quickly as you can for a block and then slow down to recover. It is that simple to do.

If you're at home with a sleeping baby and don't have the chance to get out, a jump rope is an awesome way to complete an interval training. Jump hard for a minute, then jog in place for a minute.

Or, if you have stairs in your house, you can run up the stairs and then walk back down, then run, then walk down . . .

If you don't have stairs, try doing twenty jumping jacks at full speed, then jogging in place for 30 seconds, then jumping jacks, then jogging . . . The point is, you can't convince me you can't do HIIT! Be creative and you absolutely can.

As with any form of exercise, warm up for several minutes before each workout. And please do consult your doctor before embarking on this or any exercise program.

Because of the intensity of HIIT, give yourself a day off in between. That means you should do HIIT three times per week.

So what do you on the other three days per week?

I'm a massive advocate of weight training (also known as resistance training). The reason weight training is so effective is that, like HIIT, it will raise your metabolism not just while you exercise but for hours after. It also changes your body composition, allowing you to increase your muscle mass (which helps you burn more calories) while you lose body fat.

But I understand that not everyone can get to the gym. So if you can't do weight training, then choose an activity that you love—dance, tennis, water sports, beach volleyball, or, like Krista, jumping around the house to random eighties songs. Just get active!

And here, as an added bonus, is a 20-minute workout from the phenomenal trainer to the stars Doug Kraft. He helped me lose a bunch of weight for my wedding several years ago. He's mean in the gym! (But really nice the rest of the time!)

• • • • • • • • • • • • • • • • • • • • • • • • • • • • • • • • • • • • • • • • • • • • •

## "Twenty & Plenty"

• • • • • • • • • • • • • • • • • • • • • • • • • • • • • • • • • • • • • • • • • • • • • •

### The 20 Minute Core, Cardio & Resistance Jam Session

Why 20 you ask? Twenty minutes is a good amount of time to get your heart pumping, calories burning, and muscles firing up! And why "plenty?" 'Cause it rhymes with twenty. And, as Az said, if you don't have time for a full workout, a hard 20 minutes is plenty to maximize your metabolism.

I'm keeping this simple and prop-free so no one has any excuses for not giving it all you've got. All you need is enough room to do a push-up, run in place, and perform jumping jacks. Along with that, you'll need a chair, a bench, a bed, or any flat surface a foot or two off the ground that is sturdy enough to hold your weight. Finally, you'll need a watch or a clock.

One session of Twenty & Plenty consists of the following six sets book-ended by the stretching exercises.

(Note from Krista: I just tried this workout! It's REALLY hard. You may have to do half the number of reps to begin with, then work your way up!)

### First, gently stretch to warm up

From a standing position, drop down and reach for your toes.

Next, sit with your legs flat in front of you. Lean forward and reach for your toes.

Stretch your arms by pulling each arm across your body, using your opposite hand to pull it into a stretch.

Reach your arms over your head—reach higher. Now, lean to the right, holding for a few seconds, and then lean to the left.

Okay. Now you're ready. Check the pictures if you're not sure about the form. Now load up Sue's tunes and get fired up for a hardcore Twenty & Plenty!

•   •   •   Set #1   •   •   •

**20 Push Ups!** If you need to, put your knees on the floor. Go go go!

**Jumping Jacks!** Watch the clock. Do Jumping Jacks for a full minute. Faster!

**20 Crunches!** Keep it small. Crunch it fast! Keep that heart rate up!

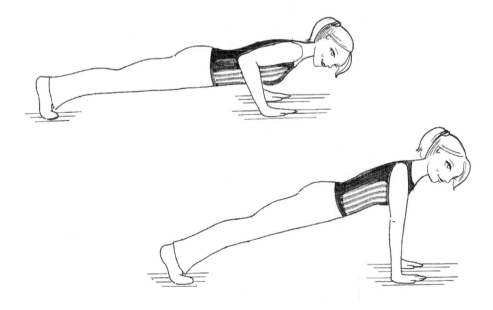

• • • **Set #2** • • •

**20 Incline Push Ups** See the picture? You can do it—go go go!

**Jumping Jacks** A full minute again

**20 More Crunches!**

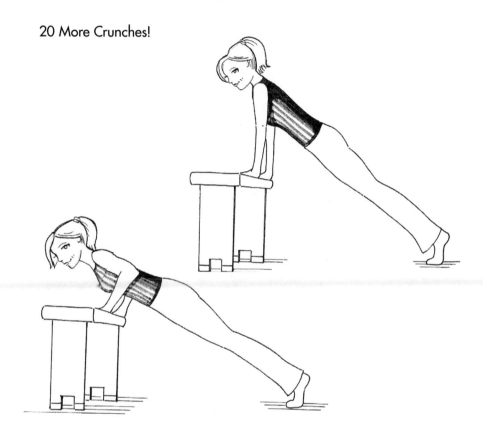

• • • **Set #3** • • •

**20 Push Ups!**

**Jumping Jacks!** Keep it up for one minute

**20 More Crunches!** Don't forget to breathe!

• • •   Set # 4   • • •

**20 Bench Ups** (these work your triceps) Look at the picture for
some guidance. Keep your back straight and your weight on your
heels! Draw in your tummy and extend your arms till they lock. It's
hard, but you can do it!

**Jumping Jacks** One minute!

**20 Bench Ups**

**Jumping Jacks** One more
minute!

**20 Bench Ups!** GO
GO GO! Don't forget
to breathe!

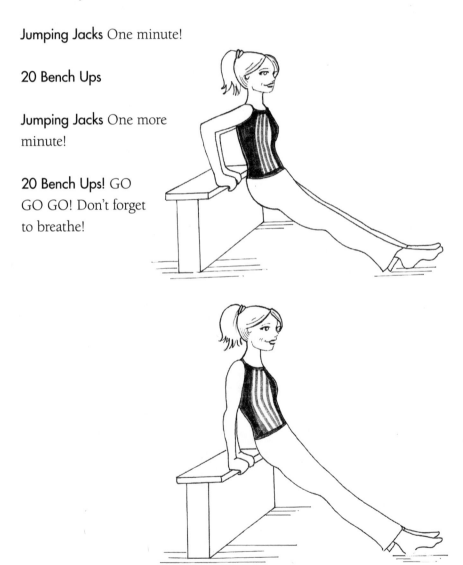

### • • • Set #5 • • •

**20 Squats!** Look at the picture then bend those legs. Take 2 seconds to bend down and two seconds to stand back up. You will feel this one in your legs tomorrow!

**Run in place** For a full minute! Knees high! Quick steady pace!

**20 More Squats**

**Run in place** For a full minute!

**20 More Squats** Feeeeeel the burn. Loooove the burn!

**Run in place** For a full minute!

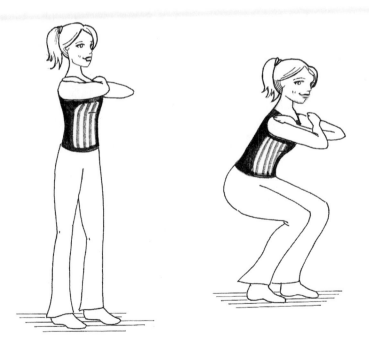

● ● ● Set #6 ● ● ●

**Boxing Punches** One full minute. See the picture? Stand in place and alternate punches one, two; one, two; one, two; quick speed, full force! Picture someone you'd like to punch!

**20 Crunches** Get back on the floor!

**Boxing Punches** Box hard for another full minute!

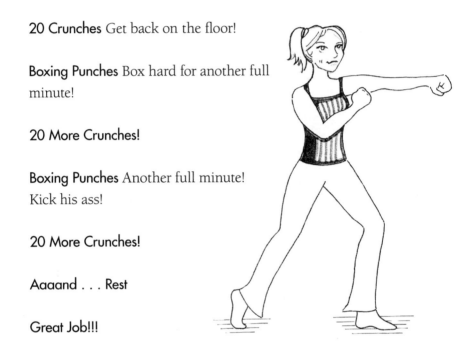

**20 More Crunches!**

**Boxing Punches** Another full minute! Kick his ass!

**20 More Crunches!**

**Aaaand . . . Rest**

**Great Job!!!**

**Make sure you stretch to cool down for a full 5 minutes!**

Sit with your legs flat in front of you. Lean forward and reach for your toes. If you're still breathing fast, keep your head high, up above your heart!

Now pull each arm across your body and use your opposite hand to pull it into a stretch.

Reach your arms over your head—reach higher. Now, lean to the right for a few seconds, before you lean to the left for a few seconds.

Keep breathing, keep working out every day, keep up your game and you will see results!

*Doug Kraft, Personal Trainer, Los Angeles, www.dougkraft.com*

● ● ● ● ● ● ● ● ● ● ● ● ● ● ● ● ● ● ● ● ● ● ● ● ● ● ●

# Frequently Asked Questions

Q: What counts as exercise?

A: Anything that speeds up your heart rate and breathing. The rule here is that you want to be able to carry on a conversation but you shouldn't be able to effectively sing a song.

Q: What if I exercise more than 20 minutes? Do I get bonus points?

A: No. You get the pride of accomplishment! You get bragging rights! You probably get quicker weight loss! But you don't get bonus points, because the game has to maintain a level playing field. You have time to exercise for more than 20 minutes. Some of your teammates and opponents may not, and we want them to have equal point-earning opportunities.

Q: What if I miss a day of exercise? Can I make it up by exercising more the next day?

A: You can make it up to your body by exercising more the next day and if you have the time and energy you absolutely should. But you can't make up the points. Those are gone forever.

Q: Whhhhhhyyyyyyy can't I make up the points???

A: Because, in case you haven't noticed, this game is all about implementing healthy habits. We are trying to get you into the HABIT of exercising every day. So stop whining. It doesn't burn nearly as many calories as you think. (Unless you are actually tantruming and stomping your feet on the floor, in which case, have at it!)

Q: What if I'm sick? Should I still exercise?

A: You have to listen to your body. Sometimes a little walking to get your blood moving or some gentle stretching will make you feel better when you're sick. And when you're sick—REALLY SICK— we allow stretching and slow walking to count as exercise. (You need not move fast enough to speed up your breathing.) But sometimes, you really just want to stay in bed. If your body is saying "Hell, no, I'm not moving!" listen to it. You will lose your exercise points for the day but you will get healthier faster and you will be able to exercise effectively sooner if you get the rest you need.

Q:   Wait. I LOSE my points if I'm too sick to exercise?? That seems totally unfair.

A:   I know. But our experience here it that it generally balances out. (E.g.: Someone on the opposing team gets sick too. Not that you should wish for that. 'Cause that would be bad karma.) And if we had a "sick rule" exception, it would be too easy to abuse. Still, if you can get out of bed and just stretch gently, that earns you full points when you're sick and may actually make you feel better. A little blood flow goes a long way.

Q:   I'm training for a marathon and running several miles a day. Why should my wife get equal points for just walking around the neighborhood?

A:   Be fair. Your wife is walking FAST around the neighborhood. Her heart rate is up; her breathing is labored (and if it's not, she should speed up). And she gets equal points because she has no time to train for a marathon, because she's too busy taking care of you, you selfish prick.

Q:   I am injured and my doctor has advised against exercise but I really want to play the game. What do I do?

A:   Ask your doctor and/or a fitness expert if there's ANY exercise you can do without further injuring yourself. If it's a leg injury, are there arm exercises you can do? Or are there physical therapy exercises you can do? If so, they count for your points. If not—if, say, you are recovering from major surgery and have been instructed to SIMPLY NOT MOVE, then talk to your teammates and opponents. Ask them to give you a task that takes 20 minutes a day and will count for your 20 exercise points. It must be something they feel will be a little hard for you but beneficial. Maybe you can write in a journal for 20 minutes a day or if you are terrible at returning e-mails or phone calls, they can assign you that task. I personally have over 15,000 e-mails in my in-box. If I were recovering from surgery, my teammates could assign me to spend 20 minutes a day organizing and deleting the e-mails in my in-box. It's not physical exercise, but it's mental exercise that would improve my life. You get the idea. Be creative. And yay you for wanting to play despite your debilitating injury. You rock.

• • • • • • • • • • • • • • • • • • • • • • • • • • • • • • • • • • • • • • • • • • • • • • • • •

## Play by the Rules

• • • • • • • • • • • • • • • • • • • • • • • • • • • • • • • • • • • • • • • • • • • • • • • • •

- Putting your body in motion for 20 minutes a day is worth 20 points a day.
- Do whatever fits into *your* life. We are not exercise snobs; just be sure to do something that makes your breath speed up.
- Take a day off.
- If serious weight-loss results are what you want, do the HIIT exercise three days a week and lift weights three days a week.
- Exercising in the morning jump-starts your metabolism, prompting you to burn more calories throughout the day.
- Exercise makes you feel good and clears your head.
- Exercise fights disease, strengthens your heart and lungs, and helps you sleep better.
- Regular exercise will increase your energy level.
- Everyone (even you) can find 20 minutes in the day to move.
- Find what motivates you and implement it into your workouts!
- Work out to fast music that you love. It really helps.

## Kevin Maynard, *lost 25 pounds*

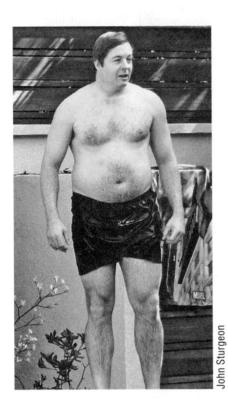

John Sturgeon

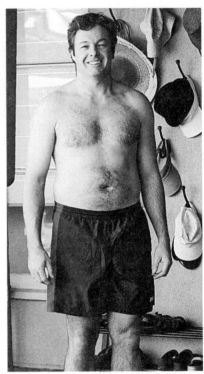

Greg Collins

I've been a jock all my life. I played hockey, football, and baseball. I skied. I ran marathons, triathlons. And until recently, I've never had a problem either putting on weight or taking it off. For me, the equation was simple—losing weight was just a matter of working out harder and longer. I do that and the pounds come off. It's a tried and true formula. But by my mid-thirties the formula had stopped working.

Pounding out ten-mile runs to take off the five pounds I'd gained during the holidays was no longer the quick fix it had been during my youth. Not only was I running more slowly now but after a week or more of inactivity, these sudden and demanding workouts would lead to a rash of hamstring and Achilles injuries. I'd need time to recover and before I knew it, that extra five pounds had ballooned into ten. Of course, in my mind, the only solution was more exercise, so I would rush through rehab, anxious to get rid of the extra weight.

That led to more injuries and more time off and now that ten pounds had become fifteen.

For years, this was my pattern. Gain weight. Work out like a madman. Get injured. I was never very worried about the weight because I knew getting rid of it was just a matter of stringing together some monster workouts. The problem was I hadn't strung together monster workouts in years.

So when Krista and Az approached me about the game I was skeptical, but I decided to give it a shot, thinking maybe I'd lose a few pounds. To date, I've lost twenty-five pounds and had a great time doing it. The simple fact is, the Game On! Diet works. And I don't get injured. I follow the plan, I play to win, and the weight comes off.

Kevin, 42

# Chapter 10

# WATER

## (Or, Are You Trying to Drown Me?)

I bought some instant water one time
but I didn't know what to add to it.

—*Steven Wright*

**The Rule:** Drink a minimum of 3 liters (about 100 ounces or 12.5 cups) of water a day for a total of 10 points each day.

**The Exception:** As with everything else, you get a day off from this rule. It does not have to be the same day off as your day off from the food plan or your day off from exercise.

**A Request:** Please consider buying a filter for your tap and refilling an aluminum or stainless steel water bottle that way. Plastic water bottles have toxins that are detrimental to your health, and the waste is severely detrimental to the health of the planet. If a filter for your tap is outside your budget, please consider a filtered pitcher. Studies show that filters create water that is at least as clean as most of what they are selling in plastic bottles!

**The biggest fight** I ever had with my husband was about how much water I drink. (I'm a water guzzler. Have been ever since I was a little kid. If you asked me, when I was seven, what my favorite drink was, I would smile smugly and say, "Water." And then all the Sprite-loving ragamuffins would glare at me with great contempt as if to say, "Are you really that big of a brownnoser?") So one night when I'm about six months pregnant and happily guzzling my water, my husband comes in and reports that he read an article about how some guy died from drinking too much water.

And I say, "Yeah, he was a marathoner and he threw off the sodium balance in his brain."

And then he says, "Yeah, but maybe you should just drink a little less."

And I laugh.

And he says, "I'm serious."

And my brain explodes.

He was basically accusing me of drowning our as-yet-unborn child. I politely screamed, *"Would you rather I drown her in crack?? How 'bout if I guzzle some nice, warm crack???"* Which made no sense but made sense to me because SERIOUSLY??? Water is my vice. WATER. I don't drink, I quit smoking, and while pregnant I was even off coffee, for God's sake. And he wants to give me crap about how much WATER I DRINK???!!!

I am not actually still mad about this. Because I got all the madness out storming around the house that night screaming about drinking crack. Still, the very best thing about being a writer? Getting the last word. In print. Hee.

Okay then, if you are feeling a little overwhelmed at the prospect of 3 liters of water a day, consider this: The very first game we played, we had to drink 4 liters of water a day and we did it and we didn't complain, so there. Fine, we complained a little. An actual e-mail from the first week:

> Az — I am drowning. I am literally drowning. I am drowning in water and I am drowning in pee. I can't go anywhere for longer than 15 minutes that doesn't have a clean toilet. Are you trying to kill me? Are you Satan? Is Hell under water?
>
> Mickey

After that, Az granted Mickey a 3-liter-a-day habit because she weighs only 120 pounds. But you know what? After a week on 4 liters, she reported that she was feeling great. Her body had adjusted to the water intake—she had tons of energy and no longer needed to pee all that much.

> My skin has NEVER been this clear. NEVER. I am shining. Glowing. If I didn't know better I'd think I was pregnant. But that would be bad 'cause I'm not big on children. I'm sticking with 4 liters.
>
> Mickey

We have settled on 3 liters (for the reasons you'll read below) but we were still experimenting in those early months of playing, and when it comes to water, some experimentation was necessary because there is so much misinformation in the press and there are so many contrasting studies.

A friend of mine called me a while back and said, hey, my newspage says there's no health benefit to drinking water! I looked on my computer and, indeed, that was the headline. Now, that wasn't exactly what the study was saying—but it sure is how it was reported. *Hey! Give up your water! Replace it with soda or booze or frothy coffee drinks! Makes no difference to your health at all!* Ummm . . . I don't want to go on a big conspiracy theory rant here, but it seems to me that it's just that kind of "report" that keeps the the big pharmaceutical companies raking in billions. Don't drink water for your headache! There's no evidence to support it! Have this pill instead! PLENTY of evidence here!!! But if you look close enough, in teeny, tiny print (or completely absent print) there's *aallll* this information about the evidence that says those pills destroy your liver and your kidneys while taking away your headache. Whatever.

While I'm on conspiracy-theory rants, I've heard the opposite one— that it's the people making billions manufacturing bottled water who want us to believe we need to hydrate. But I'm more inclined to believe that they just want us to believe we should hydrate with their particular products (many of which are not much cleaner than tap water and all of which are destroying the earth). So skip the bottled water and filter your tap water! Believe me, even if a filter seems expensive up front, you will save a ton of money in the long run by not buying bottled water!

In the end, we settled on 3 liters because it was closer to the suggestions made by the best scientific studies we could find. And what those studies come down to is this: Water is good for us. Our body is about 60 percent water so it just makes sense that water would be good for us. Water flushes toxins out of vital organs, carries nutrients to our cells, and pretty much makes every function of our bodies run more smoothly. Meanwhile, lack of water leads to dehydration (and symptoms of even *mild* dehydration include fatigue, aches, pains, headaches, dry skin, dry mouth, and just generalized misery). And not to get all gross and bathroomy about it, but every day we lose water through breath, sweat, urine, and bowel movements. In addition, heat, humidity, altitude, illness, pregnancy, breast-feeding, and certain medications all contribute to dehydration and increase our need for water. Chances are your office is heated in the winter and the weather where you live is hot in the summer. Plus, you're sweating at the gym and sweating more if you take a hot shower or bath at any point during the day. So you're losing a lot of water. Most of us lose more than we put back in. So hydrating, a lot of hydrating, is a great thing for our health.

• • • • • • • • • • • • • • • • • • • • • • • • • • • • • • • • • • • • • • • • • •

## To Spruce Up Your Water . . .

Squeeze in a splash of fresh lemon or lime juice.

Add a few organic mint leaves and several slices of cucumber.

Add the herbal tea of your choosing—my favorites are berry, citrus, or mint—and drink it hot or iced.

If you are feeling anxious, try adding chamomile tea. It's naturally sweet and has a calming effect. You can drink it hot or iced.

Do not add sweeteners to your water! Sugar is too caloric and artificial sweeteners are freaking *chemicals*. You can't put them in your body and call it water. Enjoy the herbal tea though. It's deeeelicious.

• • • • • • • • • • • • • • • • • • • • • • • • • • • • • • • • • • • • • •

And if you're in a contrary mood, and you're all, "health, shmealth, I hate health, health is stupid and I don't care," then consider this persuasive little tip from Az . . .

### • • • A Tip from Az • • •

When we don't drink enough water our bodies go into crisis mode and retain excess water, keeping some in reserves just in case things go from bad to worse. As soon as we are drinking enough water, our brains signal our bodies that the dry spell is over and our bodies respond by emptying the stores (excreting the excess fluid). That's why we all lose a bunch of weight in the first week of almost any diet or nutritional program. We gasp and say, "Wow, this diet is amazing! I lost five pounds overnight and my belly is flatter!" when all we've really done is fully hydrated ourselves.

Several years back, I trained as a Bikram yoga teacher. We did two classes a day for nine weeks. Each class was 90 to 120 minutes and the temperature was kept well above 105 degrees. By the end of the nine weeks, all the trainees' bodies were ripped. But a lot of the women were frustrated, because despite rippling muscles everywhere else, they had developed poochy bellies. It was surprising considering the intense core workouts we had done but the cute little belly bumps (which the women didn't find cute at all) could not be denied. Finally, in the week after we finished training, when those women were no longer sweating out more than they could drink, their bodies became fully hydrated and *the belly pooches disappeared.*

In addition to the cosmetic benefits, water can abate hunger pangs and give you a feeling of fullness. And a lack of water can make you feel hungry when you're really just thirsty. *So proper hydration is not only key to your health, it's key to your healthy weight loss.*

So this one's simple: For the next four weeks we're asking you to improve your health and promote healthy weight loss by choosing hydration over dehydration. Keep a full pitcher and a glass at your desk or an aluminum water bottle with you if you're on the go. Is it possible that you will drink too much water? Sure. And that may make you have to pee a couple of extra times and it may flush a few extra toxins out along the way. But it will not drown you (or your unborn child). See that? Last word.

# Frequently Asked Questions

Q:   Okay, yeah, but how much water is too much? Why did that mara-
     thoner die?

A:   Studies have been conducted in which people drank more than 2
     gallons of water a day (over 7 liters!) with no adverse effects. That
     marathoner died because he threw off the sodium balance in his
     body by dehydrating himself and then drinking *several gallons*
     of water too quickly. If you are a hardcore athlete, listen to your
     doctor's advice when it comes to sodium, electrolytes, water, and
     training.

Q:   I have heard that there are some health conditions that require
     you to limit your water intake.

A:   You're right. If you are in heart failure or suffering kidney, liver,
     or adrenal diseases, please listen to your doctor about how much
     water you should be drinking. We happily exempt you from this
     rule and wish you ever-improving health (and you can earn your
     10 water points by following your doctor's instructions as to
     proper medication/treatment each day).

Q:   Can I count my coffee/green tea/black tea/soda as water?

A:   No. We count only water and unsweetened herbal teas as water.
     Because several studies show that the caffeine, carbonation, sug-
     ars, and chemical sweeteners in other beverages can have detri-
     mental effects. And this is our tricky little way of encouraging you
     to drink less of those other beverages. (Three liters of water doesn't
     leave you thirsty for much else.) By the way, no soda is allowed
     while playing the game except on your day off and meal off! This
     includes diet soda!!

Q:   I like my sleep and I don't want to be up all night peeing. What do
     I do?

A:   Finish drinking all your water at least two hours before bedtime.
     There's a school of thought in traditional Chinese medicine that

says drinking a liter of warm water upon awakening will keep your bowels moving regularly and awaken your organs for the day. So maybe try that—that way you have a whole liter out of the way first thing in the morning!

Q: Do I get extra points if I drink more than 3 liters?

A: No, point hog, you don't.

Q: If I miss a liter one day, can I drink 4 the next day and get my points back?

A: Nope. This game is about, among other things, becoming present and conscious about your health habits. I am SO a person who would like to be able to do 2 liters one day and 4 the next because I tend to be pretty disorganized. But the game requires me to pay more attention and paying more attention seems to be a key to health and weight loss. That said, we do allow you a day off from this rule. And you can take your day off any day of the week. So if on Thursday morning you wake up and realize you didn't drink all your water on Wednesday, you can call Wednesday your water day off and not lose any points! Aren't we nice?

## Play by the Rules

- Drink a minimum of 3 liters of water a day to earn 10 points a day.
- You get one day off from the water rule.
- Feel free to drink extra water, but you don't get extra points.
- If you miss a liter, you can't make it up the next day.
- Please buy a refillable water bottle—ideally, an aluminum or stainless steel one—and a water filter (so as not to destroy the planet).
- If you feel like you're drowning in the first few days, stick with it; your body will adjust.

## Chapter 11

# SLEEP

### (Or, Shhhhhhhzzzzzzzzzzzzzz...)

Sleeping is no mean art:
for its sake one must stay awake all day.

—*Friedrich Nietzsche*

> **The Rule:** To earn your 15 sleep points, you must be in bed with the lights out a minimum of seven hours before you know you have to wake up.
>
> **The Exception:** If you suffer from severe insomnia—severe enough that you have been to see at least one doctor or specialist about your inability to fall asleep or stay asleep—then you can earn your 15 sleep points each day by practicing at least three of the sidebar suggestions from the National Sleep Foundation each night or by practicing the bedtime yoga routine described at the end of this chapter.

**Here's what happens** when my baby doesn't get her requisite eleven hours of sleep a night—like, say, when I have to wake her up early because we have a plane to catch.

First, she wakes up screaming at the top of her lungs.

Then, she looks at me with great sadness in her eyes, mixed with a hearty dose of confusion and a smidge of betrayal. It's a look that says, "What in the hell is wrong with you, woman? Fork over the boob juice and let's get some shut-eye!" Then there's the frantic kicking of legs as I bring her to the table to change her diaper. She kicks as if she believes that if she kicks hard enough, water will magically appear and she will swim back to the warm comfort of bed.

When I finally get her dressed and into the car, she usually forgives me because (a) she kinda likes the car and (b) she really likes her dad, who is, by this time, sitting beside her roaring like Frankenstein to make her laugh.

Still, our sleep-deprived baby will then spend the morning alternately weepy and frenetic—say, repeatedly trying to grab the hair of the passenger in the seat in front of us on the plane and shrieking with outrage when we pull her out of reach. Fun!

When I haven't had enough sleep, my head hurts, I feel nauseated, and I crave baked goods. (Prior to knowing Az, I subscribed wholeheartedly to the theory that airport calories don't count. Because you're tired when you travel. And when you're tired you stop at Starbucks. And no God I want to believe in would punish you in any way for adding a delightful scone to soak up some of your highly caffeinated beverage. Sadly, Az disagreed.) When I'm sleep deprived, I also can't think as clearly, can't write as well, and can't help but feel overwhelmed rather than delighted by my fun job and my beautiful baby. I also pick fights with my husband and am unfriendly to my cats.

A lack of sleep affects every aspect of my day—so why am I, why are we, as a culture, so inclined to prioritize everything else above our sleep? When did we learn to stop crying and kicking and wailing about it? Wouldn't it be awesome if the next time your boss asked you to come in too early, you just burst into tears and screamed, "WHYYYYYYYYYYYY???" Or if, the next time your friends invited you for a dinner party on a Friday night when they know you will have just wrapped up a sixty-hour work week, you just started kicking them repeatedly? "Don't (kick) you know (kick) I'm TIRED (kick kick kick)??!!!"

When Az added the sleep rule to the game, my friend Jana threatened to quit. She's a working mother of two and the idea of trying to force herself to stay in bed for seven hours when she "feels perfectly fine on less than six" was appalling to her. But I bullied her into playing. I was all, "Chiiicken. Bock bock—bock bock. Whatsa matter? You afraid of a little sleeeeep?" Then she was all, "Screw you! Game on, Fatty." (Heh. The written version of my friendships are so much meaner than in actual life. In actual life I probably said, "Come on, honey, just play, and if you lose some sleep points, it'll be all right." And she said, "Okay." But how boring is that?)

Well wouldn't you know it? Jana came around. An actual e-mail from her:

You know how much I hated this rule? Well, it has improved my entire life. I thought I was fine on six hours, but apparently I was cranky and unpleasant on six hours. Didn't even know it. I feel better, happier, stronger, and my kids and husband like me more. Plus I'm getting better workouts and am no longer planning that post-office shooting. Kidding about the shooting. But honestly love the rule. And the sleep. LOVE the sleep.

Jana

So, I say, sleep more. But in addition to my opinion, there are actual medical and biological reasons for this rule, too. According to the latest studies, healthy sleep is the single most important factor in predicting longevity. Seriously, it's more important than diet, exercise, or heredity!

## The Detrimental Effects of Sleep Deprivation on Health and Weight Loss Include:

- Weakened immune system
- Increased carbohydrate cravings
- Decreased alertness and ability to focus
- Increased risk of depression and irritability
- Increased body weight
- Decreased ability to react
- Increased risk of cancer, diabetes, heart disease
- Increased risk of obesity
- Increased bitchiness
- Increased risk of nodding off during sex

So, yeah, as it turns out, healthy sleep is not a luxury.

I'm guessing that some of you are reading this right now and thinking that this chapter doesn't apply to you. Like Jana, you think you're different. You think you require less sleep. I'm guessing you think this because in study after study, researchers have found that *most Americans* believe they are getting enough sleep at six hours. We believe, despite mountains of evidence to the contrary, that our bodies have "adjusted" to getting less sleep and that we are "fine." We say we're fine but then we go to the doctor for antibiotics for endless infections; we suffer flu, muscle stiffness, and aches and pains; we buy diet supplements to counter our carb cravings; we go to physical therapists to recover from injuries caused by "clumsy" accidents and to psychiatrists for mood-improving pharmaceuticals. And the thing is? It's all connected.

There's really good science to support the idea that we are *not fine* on less than seven to eight hours of sleep. We are sick because we are tired. We are clumsy because we are tired. We are irritable and depressed and anxious, and often, it's *because we're tired.* And if that weren't enough, there's a growing body of evidence that suggests that we are FAT because we are tired. Okay, we also eat too much and don't exercise enough. But part of why we eat too much and don't exercise enough is that we're TIRED.

The best sleep research concludes that seven to eight hours a night is a healthy amount of sleep for most people (less than 5 percent of the population can thrive on seven hours or less), which means *almost everyone has accrued a sleep debt which should be repaid.*

• • • • • • • • • • • • • • • • • • • • • • • • • • • • • • • • • • • • •

## Are You in Sleep Debt?

Do you require caffeine to wake up in the morning?

Is it hard for you to wake up in the morning despite getting a good night's sleep?

Do you constantly hit "snooze" when your alarm goes off?

Do you get sleepy in the middle of your workday?

Are you able to nap easily?

If you answered yes to ANY of these questions, you are very likely in sleep debt. The good news is, you can pay it back at any time!

• • • • • • • • • • • • • • • • • • • • • • • • • • • • • • • • • • • • •

Now, please don't think for a minute that I'm judging. I am not standing on the outside of this one, all lofty and high and mighty and healthy and whole. I'm a coffee girl. Loooove my coffee. Love it so much that despite having been told by more than one allergist that I am *allergic to it,* I drink it every day. Apparently, in addition to my highly addictive personality, my coffee habit may also have something to do with my sleep debt.

Hmmm . . . Y'think?? I have a fifteen-month-old! And a job! And I'm writing a book about playing a game, for God's sake. When am I supposed to sleep???

The answer, apparently, is whenever I can. Naps are good. Naps help. Also, sleeping in whenever you can helps. The debt is like a bank debt—if you're running a negative balance, then any time you can put a few dollars in, you're gaining ground. And here's a thing to think about: When we run a negative bank account balance, we do a lot of things to address the situation. We work more hours, get second jobs, cut back on our spending . . . So with all this research telling us that we are in the throes of serious sleep debt and that it is wreaking havoc on our physical health and emotional well-being, what are we willing to change to address the situation? Work fewer hours? Quit the second job? Cut back on our social lives? It sounds impossible, doesn't it? It sounds crazy.

It's a societal plague, this notion we've all adopted that sleep is not only inessential but detrimental to true effectiveness. "You snooze, you lose." "I'll sleep when I'm dead." "The early bird catches the worm." No wonder it sounds wrong that we're asking you to prioritize your sleep for the next four weeks.

The good news is, studies have shown that once the sleep debt is repaid, the vast majority of people will naturally fall into a rhythm of seven to eight hours a night. For this reason, the game doesn't put a limit on how much sleep you can get; it puts a limit only on how *little* sleep you can get.

Seven hours. Minimum. (And the fact is, you REALLY SHOULD be getting eight, so we're already giving you a break.)

### Step Up Your Game!

If you are already in the habit of getting seven hours of sleep a night, make a commitment to yourself and your team that you will get a minimum of eight hours of sleep a night or you lose your sleep points. See how that extra hour improves your whole life!

Fifteen points is a lot, yeah. But it's a lot for a reason. Sleep. Sleep more. Sleep a lot more and see how your life improves. Our culture may call you lazy but the game is giving you carte blanche to call it a night at 8 p.m. Admit it. You're kind of excited. 'Cause what's better than guilt-free sleep? Nothing, that's what.

•  •  •  •  •  •  •  •  •  •  •  •  •  •  •  •  •  •  •  •  •  •  •  •  •  •  •  •  •  •  •  •

Suffering from insomnia? You're not alone. If you are one of the millions of Americans with a diagnosed sleep disorder and are therefore *unable* to go to sleep for seven hours straight to earn your points, then you can earn your points by trying the following suggestions from the National Sleep Foundation. You must try three a week and you must do all three consistently every night of the week to earn all your sleep points. (By the way, the following tips are great for everyone, whether you suffer from a sleep disorder or not!)

1.  Maintain a regular bedtime and wake-time schedule, including weekends. Our sleep-wake cycle is regulated by a circadian clock in our brain and by the body's need to balance both sleep time and wake time. Regular bedtimes at night and waking times in the morning strengthen the circadian function and can help you fall asleep at night and wake up refreshed in the morning.

2.  Establish a regular, relaxing bedtime routine, such as soaking in a hot bath or hot tub and then reading a book or listening to soothing music. Avoid bright lights and arousing activities before bedtime. No working, paying bills, engaging in competitive games, or family problem-solving for at least two hours before you try to go to sleep.

3.  Create a sleep-conducive environment that is dark, quiet, comfortable, and cool. Consider using blackout curtains, eye shades, ear plugs, "white noise" (like an alarm clock with a rainforest setting), humidifiers, fans, and other devices. Dry is bad. Hot is bad. And a partner who snores? Sooo bad. If your partner snores and your earplugs don't do the trick, try sleeping in another room. (It's not ideal but it beats perpetual sleep deprivation.)

4.  Sleep on a comfortable mattress and pillows. Make sure your

mattress is comfortable and supportive. The one you have been using for years may have exceeded its life expectancy—about nine or ten years for most good-quality mattresses. Yes, a new mattress is a serious financial investment, but you spend a third of your life in bed. So if you know you need a new mattress and you can't afford it, start saving for one. Even a few bucks a day adds up. (Y'know, that few bucks a day you spend on coffee to recover from your crappy night's sleep.)

5. Use your bedroom only for sleep and sex. Take work materials, cell phones, computers, and televisions out of the bedroom! Low lighting, aromatherapy, and quiet music (and maybe some good sex before bed) all help.

6. Finish eating at least two to three hours before your regular bedtime. Consider eliminating spices from your last meal to avoid heartburn. Also, try to finish all your water at least two hours before bed so you don't wake up a lot to pee. Chamomile tea is an exception. You might try some before bed to quiet your mind and calm your nerves.

7. Exercise regularly but complete your workout at least a few hours before bedtime. During exercise, body temperature rises—making you more alert—and takes as long as six hours to start dropping. A cooler body temperature is associated with sleep onset. Late afternoon exercise is the perfect way to help you fall asleep at night.

8. Avoid caffeine (e.g., coffee, caffeinated tea, soft drinks, chocolate). Caffeine is a stimulant; that's why we love it. Caffeine stays in the body on average from three to five hours, but can affect some people *up to twelve hours later.* So if you have trouble sleeping, either quit caffeine completely or avoid it for at least eight hours before going to bed!

9. Avoid nicotine. Used close to bedtime, it can lead to poor sleep. Nicotine is also a stimulant. Smoking before bed makes it more difficult to fall asleep. In addition, when smokers go to sleep, they experience withdrawal symptoms from nicotine, which also cause sleep problems. Difficulty sleeping: just one more reason to quit smoking. Also, the cancer. Just saying.

10. Avoid alcohol close to bedtime. Although many people think of

alcohol as a sedative, it actually disrupts sleep, causing nighttime awakenings. Consuming alcohol leads to a night of less restful sleep. Not to mention, it leads to massive point losses in the game! If you are in the habit of having a drink to relax before bed, replace that ritual with 10 minutes of gentle stretching and 5 minutes or more of quiet meditation.

• • • • • • • • • • • • • • • • • • • • • • • • • • • • • • • • • • • • • • • • • •

## A word from yogini Jennifer Bloom
## Undress Your Stress

*You take off your heels and jeans before bed, right? You should probably shed some tension, too. Sneak in these three yoga techniques right before bedtime and give your body a head start on relaxing into sleep.*

1. **Lay on the Floor First.** *Not the bed, the floor. Lay on your back, arms out, palms up, either with your legs out long or with your knees up and soles of the feet down. Let gravity work together with the firmness of the floor to gently release all the little kinks in the small of your back and between your shoulder blades. Take ten deep, slow breaths.*

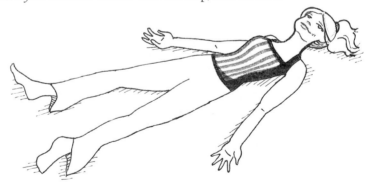

2. **Neck Release.** *Try a modified rabbit pose: Sitting on the edge of your bed with your knees apart, interlace your fingers behind your back, and puff out your heart and chest by drawing your shoulders back. Now fold at the waist, and drop your head between your knees, allowing your arms and combined fist to fall forward over your head. Breathe into the space between the shoulder blades as you shake your head yes and no, and feel*

*the tension practically drip off
your head.*

3. **Goddess Hips.** *Most of us cross
our legs or sit knees together for
most of the day, accumulating a
lot of stress around the hips and
pelvis. This is not good! (Especially if you're trying to encourage toxins and cellulite to move
out of this area.) Once you
get into bed, lay on your back,
open your knees wide, and bring the
soles of your feet together. Place your
hands on your belly and breathe as low
into the pelvis as you can.
It might feel awkward at
first, like a frog awaiting
dissection, but even-
tually your hips will
relax, and your
dreams at night
will be full of abundance
and life.*

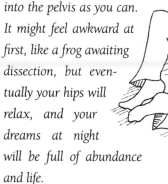

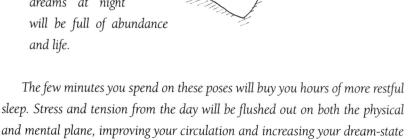

*The few minutes you spend on these poses will buy you hours of more restful
sleep. Stress and tension from the day will be flushed out on both the physical
and mental plane, improving your circulation and increasing your dream-state
creativity.*

*Good night!*

*—Jennifer Bloom, yoga teacher and healer*
*www.yogablooms.com*

# Frequently Asked Questions

Q:  Number one on the Sleep Foundation list is go to sleep at the same time every night and wake up at the same time every morning. But you seem to be suggesting that in order to repay my sleep debt I should go to bed early and sleep late whenever I can. 'Splain, please?

A:  Once your sleep debt is paid, it's a great idea to go to bed and wake up at the same time every night and morning—even on weekends. But just like the banker wants his bucks back, your body wants its sleep back. Until you are awake and alert throughout the day, never craving naps or nodding at your desk in the afternoon, grab extra Z's when you can. A possible exception to this is insomniacs who have a very hard time falling asleep at night. If you are an insomniac, try the same time every night and morning thing and see if it helps you actually get to sleep more easily.

Q:  If I have trouble falling asleep, can I just take a sleeping pill?

A:  Even if you aren't a diagnosed insomniac, you will benefit from the Sleep Foundation suggestions. We all want a quick fix so we run to the doctor for sleeping pills while chugging back grande lattes and watching action movies in bed. Before you turn to pharmaceuticals (which can be addictive and detrimental to your health in other ways), try the suggestions from the Sleep Foundation. Also consider trying natural alternatives to pharmaceuticals (chamomile tea, aromatherapy, valerian root).

Q:  What if I wake up in the middle of the night and can't get back to sleep? Do I lose my points?

A:  No. We don't require you to be ASLEEP for seven hours to earn your points. That would only create anxiety, which would interfere with your sleep. We are asking you to be in bed with the light out and your eyes closed seven hours before you know you have to be up. If you are inclined to lie in bed wide awake and THINK for hours, the National Sleep Foundation recommends that you get up and try meditation or deep breathing. You'll be amazed how effective it can be in helping you get more better-quality sleep. If you need to do this, you will still earn your points.

Q:  I am a new parent. My baby wakes me up every hour or two all night long. I can go to sleep seven hours before the baby's up for the day, but I sure won't be getting seven hours of sleep. How do I earn my points?

A:  Specialists suggest that you go to sleep a minimum of eight and ideally nine or ten hours before you know your baby will be up for the day. It will make you a happier parent and that will make for a happier baby! So consider committing to yourself and your team that you will be in bed a minimum of eight hours before you know you will have to be up for the day. It's hard but it's possible and it's the very best thing you can do for yourself, your baby, your relationship, and your sanity. Go you!

Q:  I work odd hours and cannot possibly get seven hours sleep in a row. How do I earn my points?

A:   If it is literally impossible for you to get seven hours of sleep without quitting your job, you can take your sleep in shifts and still earn your points. BUT—you should consider committing to get at least eight hours total sleep to earn your points. (The extra hour is to compensate for the compromised quality of sleep taken in shifts.)

## Play by the Rules

- Seven hours of sleep (preferably eight) equals 15 points.
- Almost every person needs seven to eight hours of sleep.
- Adequate sleep will prolong your life with your new healthy body.
- Inadequate sleep affects you physically, emotionally, and psychologically.

- Lack of sleep weakens your immune system and makes you more susceptible to getting sick.
- When you are tired, you crave carbohydrates.
- Lack of sleep makes you cranky and no fun to be around. Not to mention accident-prone.
- If you are in sleep debt, take naps and sleep whenever you can until you catch up.
- When you eliminate your sleep debt, your body will thank you and naturally fall into a rhythm of seven to eight hours a night.
- If you suffer from insomnia or are having trouble sleeping, please refer to the sidebar in this chapter for some helpful tips.

Chapter 12

# TRANSFORMATION

### (Or, Habits? That's, Like, Nun's Clothes, Right?)

Nothing so needs reforming
as other people's habits.

—*Mark Twain*

> **The Rule:** You earn 10 points a day by eliminating an unhealthy habit and 10 points a day by practicing a new healthy habit. You must declare you habit choices to your teammates and stick with them for the entire game.
>
> **The Penalty:** Each time you change your habit choices, you lose 50 points, so choose carefully!
>
> **The Exception:** You get a day off from this rule too—but be smart about it. If you are quitting smoking or something similar, don't take a day off or you'll destroy your progress.

**Truth be told,** this is the part that intrigued me most when Az first proposed the game. Sure, I was sort of sick of my expanding waistline, but I was happily married with a wonderful baby and a reasonable clothing budget that allowed me to buy ever-bigger clothes that didn't cling. I also have a very vivid imagination that allowed me to believe that clothes were just being made smaller and that I was not actually at a size that required me to shop in the plus-size section of Nordstrom's. I *was* shopping in the plus-size section of Nordstrom's—I just refused to believe that I *had* to. I was all, "This is just more *comfortable.* I like loose, flowy things. It's *hot* in California. I'm not actually *this big.*" So, yeah, I was intrigued with the diet and exercise part of the game, but this habit part? It's the thing that made me really want to play.

Az's actual original e-mail to me:

Dear Krista,

I challenge you to a fitness game. It will be played for points. You and Jana and Mickey against me and Anselm and Kevin. Boys vs Girls. We will compete for tickets to a show in Vegas—winner's choice. We will win points for food and

water and exercise. Plus we all have to take on one bad habit we'd like to eliminate and one good habit we'd like integrate into our lives. We'll get points for all
of it, we'll play for nine weeks, and the team with the most points wins.

Cheers,

Az

You heard me. Nine weeks. NINE. He sent me a casual e-mail proposing
that I DIET COMPETITIVELY for NINE WEEKS. So here's how I read it:

Dear Chunker,

I challenge your tubby ass that keeps asking me for diet advice but won't actually do what I say to a game. Because you have been known to make people
cry with your competitive ranting on Games Nights, maybe this will get your
blubbery butt on the stationary bike. Because you LOATHE to lose, you will be
FORCED to do what I say—e.g.: eat kibble and drink toilet water—or risk losing
for you and your team. HA! This will be AWESOME (for me. You will hate it). Oh,
and you'll get to take on some of your habits, which you might actually enjoy
and which might take your mind off the kibble-eating.

Cheers,

Az

For the record and just in case you haven't read the food chapter
yet, there was no kibble-eating. I lost more than fifteen pounds in that
nine weeks and it wasn't painful and it was actually fun. The next time
we played, I was excited to go back on the food plan and lose more
weight. But the *first* time I played, it was the transformation points that
hooked me.

I like the idea that people can change. That "old dogs, new tricks"
adage bugs the crap out of me. It has been my experience and my observation that when it comes to changing, age is a benefit. As we grow older,
we know ourselves better, and we can and should use that self-knowledge
to continue to evolve. My dad went to law school at the age of forty-seven.
This was a man who didn't have a college education but did have a brilliant

mind. It just took him nearly fifty years to grow up enough that he wanted to use it. He persuaded the college to acknowledge his life experience and give him an undergrad degree for it. And then he took on law school. The number of habits and routines he had to change to make it work was tremendous. He struggled, no doubt. But at fifty, he graduated law school near the top of his class, with high honors. Old dogs, new tricks, my ass.

Don't worry. We're not asking you to go to law school. We're just asking you to take a look at your habits—all of your habits, not just the obvious ones—and pick one you'd like to be rid of and pick one you'd like to add.

Only you know what you really need and want to change in your life. Note that I said need *and* want—because the want part is the key. Many people—family, friends, doctors—bitched at me for many years to quit smoking, but I didn't do it successfully till my dad died of esophageal cancer at fifty-six. At his death bed, I promised him I would quit. He didn't ask me to—he couldn't talk by that point—but I wanted to offer him something. I wanted him to know before he left that some small good thing might come from the horrible mess he had made of his own body. And then, I wanted to honor the promise, so after a few weeks of chain-smoking to assuage the grief, I did.

Smoking is an obvious one. If you are reading this book, and you are still smoking . . . I'm not judging. I'm just saying that this game is about optimizing your health and smoking does quite the opposite. So I hope you quit. I even hope you use the game to quit. I have two friends, Ray and Corey, who did just that!

*I cannot believe I've gone four weeks without a cigarette. I really can't believe it. I have been a closet smoker for eleven years—eleven years, every day, sneaking cigarettes like a junkie on the make. And now I haven't had a single one in twenty-eight days. AND I haven't gained weight, which was my big fear. I was all, "I can live with black lung, just not a beer gut." And now I don't have either. I love it! The game rocks. I thank you, my lungs thank you, and my dogs, who are no longer doomed to an early death from secondhand smoke poisoning, thank you.*

*—Corey, 36*

Smoking aside, here are a few other habits you might consider.

**Drugs:** Maybe you are using some illegal drugs that you know aren't good for you. Or maybe you are using some prescription drugs that you know you don't need. Either way, give them up for four weeks and watch how your life changes. You might be surprised. (If you take this on, please consult a doctor first!)

**Complacency:** If you give up complacency, you must specify what you mean. E.g.: Once an hour, I will get up from my desk and walk all around the perimeter of the office. Or, I will do three Sun Salutations a day. Or, I will walk or bike to work instead of driving. Be specific!

**Lying:** This is a big one. If you catch yourself lying, even a small lie, you must correct the lie with the person you lied to or lose your points for the day!

**Negative self-talk:** Most of us speak unkindly to ourselves several times throughout the day. Each time you catch it, you must take the time to rethink—e.g.: *I'm not a fat bastard. I'm a good guy and I'm working hard to change what isn't working.* If you don't stop and rethink, you lose your points for the day.

**Cursing:** Maybe you have a kid now? And she's started picking up on your potty mouth? And you don't want her to grow up going, "Pass the fucking block this way, Jakie!"? Consider this: Each time a curse word comes out of your mouth, you will lose your points or put $5 in a jar, then at the end of the game, you'll donate the contents to Habitat for Humanity or the charity of your choice (and the charity can't be you). By the end of the game, you'll have broken the cursing habit or gone broke for a good cause!

**Coffee:** If you are drinking, like, eight cups a day, don't quit cold turkey. Set a plan that goes something like three cups a day for week 1, two cups for week 2, one cup for week 3, then for week 4 . . . Oy. If you can give it up entirely and stay sane and functional, you have my utmost respect. Be warned: You may suffer headaches as you begin to withdraw— try to get a little extra sleep and drink some extra water to help with the withdrawal symptoms.

**Texting while driving:** This is a fatal practice. FATAL. You wouldn't drink and drive. And if you are in the habit of texting and driving, please take this on and quit cold turkey!

**Watching TV** (except *Grey's Anatomy*—don't give up *Grey's Anatomy*): Turn it off. Or commit to only one hour a night. You'll be amazed at how much time you suddenly have!

**Mindlessly surfing the Internet:** Same as TV. This is where all your time is going! Give yourself a half hour to play online and that's it.

**Video games:** Same as TV and the Internet. These are a HUGE time-suck.

**Internet porn:** Turn it off. You'll be amazed at how much more respect you suddenly have for women. And farm animals.

**Gossip:** Make the commitment that you won't say anything behind anyone's back that you wouldn't say to his or her face. If you slip, you have to stop the minute you catch yourself and say three kind things about the person and make an earnest wish or say a prayer for his or her success and happiness or lose your points. This can be time-consuming—and eventually, you'll break the unconscious habit. As an added bonus, you'll worry less that people are trash-talking you!

**Watching the news:** Turning off the news for a month has TREMEN-DOUS benefits for your health and well-being! Televised news is as negative as they can make it. It's designed to scare you and studies show it prompts serious anxiety. Quit it like a bad drug. Read the news instead. Better yet, read it only one day a week. Because the human psyche was not designed to take in all the bad news of the world every day of the week. Stay informed—just with less frequency. You'll be *amazed* at how much better you feel.

**Ordering in:** If you are in the habit of ordering in even one meal a day, you would be startled by the effect that giving it up has on the planet. The southern U.S. remains the world's largest paper-producing region and every year millions of acres of the South's forest are cleared to feed the pulp and paper industry. So give up one meal and you're helping to save the Southern forests right here in the United States. Or consider this juggernaut of a statistic: If we all used *one fewer napkin a day,* more than a billion pounds of napkins could be saved from landfills each year. Take this on. You'll be doing us all a favor!

**Buying bottled water:** If you are buying bottled water every day, giving it up for four weeks will save energy, oil, and landfill space. "Approximately 1.5 million barrels of oil—enough to run 100,000 cars for a whole year—are used to make plastic water bottles, while transporting these bottles burns even more oil . . . In addition to the millions of gallons of water used in the plastic-making process, two gallons of water are wasted in the purification process for every gallon that goes into the bottles" (www.treehugger.com).

Get a refillable bottle and a filter for your tap water. It's not expensive when you consider what you're spending on bottled water. After a week or two, you'll actually be saving a lot of money! If you go to www.thegame ondiet.com, you can buy a refillable aluminum water bottle and we will give all the proceeds to the Environmental Defense Fund.

The habit I took on that first game out? TV. (Ironic, right?) But here's the thing: I complain a lot about not having time to do all the things I want in this life. I want to become a better guitar player. I want to learn a foreign language. I want to be better about keeping in touch with old friends. I want to do yoga, learn to like to meditate, keep a journal. I want more quality time with my husband, more time to read really good books, more time with my friends, more sleep. And I always feel like I just don't have enough time for any of it. Except . . . I watch HOURS of TV every night. At least two hours. Sometimes three. Occasionally four.

So I asked myself, if I limited my TV-viewing to one hour a night, what would happen to my life? Well, I tried it. And what happened is . . . I was incredibly irritated for several days and simply went to sleep early because I was too annoyed about missing *So You Think You Can Dance* to stay awake.

But that was just the first few days. After that, what happened is that I had time to do—and I DID—every single thing on the above list. (Okay, I didn't learn a language. But I swear, I had so much time, I could have.) I practiced my guitar every day. I wrote to old friends, had dinner with others, did yoga, seriously contemplated meditating (MAN, do I struggle with meditating), read great books, and got plenty of sleep (and frankly, I slept better). I never realized what a massive time-suck TV was in my life until I turned it off.

Maybe TV isn't your thing. Maybe for you, like my husband, it's sports. I swear the man can spend an entire day checking sports Web sites, reading sports magazines, watching sports TV—and then complain that he has no time.

Almost everyone I know has a version of this. Like gossip. I have friends—and by friends I mean me—who can spend HOURS talking about the lives of other people. To what end? To what gain? All that gossiping does for me is make me paranoid that it's being done *to me*. It doesn't make me a better person, and in some cases, it can actually be harmful. So, it's another one I've worked on while playing the game. Honestly, it's the hardest one I've worked on and I lost a lot of points that game, but I did get more mindful of the words coming out of my mouth, so I considered it a successful experiment. Which brings me to an observation I've made in all my months of playing this game: The more extreme habits—the ones that are more likely to kill us—are sometimes easier to change.

In my adult life, I have quit drinking and quit smoking successfully. But when I tried to quit gossiping, I was less successful. I think in part because there is a TON of support from family and friends when you decide you're ready to quit smoking. But when you decide to quit gossiping? People look at you suspiciously and call you boring to your face. When you turn off your TV? You feel utterly left out of water-cooler conversations, plus, people call you boring to your face. So the benefits of giving up the habit you choose have to outweigh the losses—because there will be losses.

> *At the beginning of the game, I started writing down every time I judged my body and I was horrified—there were days I would say "You're fat" to myself twenty-five times. I thought,* Imagine if I said that to my child! *By forcing myself to rethink each time, I broke the habit and I can't express how good it feels.*
>
> —Duffy, 39

Do you have to be extreme in your choice of which habit to give up? No. Can you start small? Like, one fewer hour of TV a night? Yes. But I will tell you from experience that the benefit to your life will be directly proportional to how big you go. Turn off the TV completely for a month and your life will improve radically compared with turning it off an hour early. And yet, turning it off an hour early is no small feat, and if that's what you've got in you, then that's what you should do. Just pick a thing. Pick a thing you want to change, declare it to your teammates, and change it. Don't panic. It's just four weeks. (Unless you like the change so much, you keep it for a lifetime. How cool would that be?)

> *Whenever I ate or drank something in the evening I would always put my glass or dish in the sink and expect my wife to rinse it off and put it in the dishwasher. For my good habit, I decided to start rinsing off those evening dishes and put them in the dishwasher myself. Now, even though the game's over, I still do that. And my wife appreciates it. I'm not sure if I'm getting more sex because of it, but I'm a better husband for it.*
>
> —Mark, 50

Which brings us to part 2: *choosing a new habit* . . .

You know all the things I listed above as things I don't have time for? All good habits that I would like to integrate into my life. Feel free to pick from that list or to pick one of your own. The idea here is that you are trying to integrate a healthy habit. It's something you are going to do every day for the next twenty-eight days. Make it a challenge—but it doesn't have to be time-consuming (if time is a limitation in your life). For example, a few games back, I chose flossing. I know. At thirty-six, I needed to force myself to floss my teeth every night and I'm admitting to it in print. But that's because I'm pretty sure I'm not the only one. And I'm pretty happy with the fact that since that game ended, I've kept up the habit completely. And my dentist and hygienist? Freaked out last week when I went for my check up. They were like a tooth paste commercial, they were so excited. Apparently, it makes a big difference. So yay me.

Pick something that will improve your life or will improve your health or will make you feel better about yourself and the world on a daily basis. Whether it's flossing your teeth, or practicing piano for 20 minutes a day, or reading for half an hour every night, or giving thanks every night, or stretching before bed, or . . . or . . . or . . . You know what you need in your life. Pick a thing and stick to it for twenty-eight days and see what happens.

## Some Common Healthy Habit Choices

- Take up cooking (at least one meal a day).
- Organize your house or clear clutter.
- Study a foreign language.
- Learn or practice a musical instrument.
- Rediscover reading for pleasure.
- Take up journaling.
- Take up yoga.
- Take up meditation.
- Floss daily.
- Call three people you like each day.
- Be of service to others. (Do charitable work.)

The habits may seem small but the commitment to change is big. Think carefully about your options, because we are asking you to pick them once (one new habit you are integrating, one old habit you are quitting) and *stick to them for the whole game.*

You can do it. You rock. Yay you.

## Frequently Asked Questions

Q: What if I chose poorly? Can I change my choice?

A: "Chose poorly" generally means that you chose *hard* and are struggling and feel you are losing too many points for your team. So before you change, consider why you chose the habit you did. Chances are it's because it's a thing you really do need to work on in your life. Can you work a little harder on it? Can you stick with it for one more week? Can you recommit?? Consider trying harder before you change—because you *lose 50 points* every time you change a declared habit. We impose this rule for a reason. According to researchers, it takes twenty-eight days to successfully change a habit for life. If you change yours after a week or two, you aren't getting the full benefit of the challenge.

**Q:** Okay, yeah, but have you ever changed a habit mid-game?

**A:** Yes. I tried to give up coffee once. I wanted to kill myself. I couldn't do my job or write this book or function. Which tells me that I am truly addicted to the stuff and really should consider actually quitting it some time. Maybe slowly cut back until I'm off it completely. But I didn't declare that I was cutting back. I took it on cold turkey, and I failed failed failed. But I learned a lot from the attempt, so all was not lost. However, 50 points were lost—50 POINTS. IT SUUUUUUUCKS to lose 50 points. So again, choose carefully.

**Q:** Does it have to be a "bad" habit, or can it just be something that I want to change in my life?

**A:** It can just be something you want to change. And feel free to be creative. One game, I wanted to floss my teeth as my new habit but I also wanted to make sure I stretched for 20 minutes each day. So my new habit choice was flossing, and the thing I decided to let go of was complacency. Worked nicely.

**Q:** If I can't think of any habits that I want to change, can I help my husband change his bad habits?

**A:** Heh. Hee hee. I like your thinking. But no. What you could do is take a look at your own control issues. You could try giving up expressing any opinions about anyone else's life for four weeks. See how that goes. I bet it's tough for you. (I know it would be for me.)

**Q:** If I have a big project that I have been avoiding, like cleaning my garage, will it count if I do a little bit each day?

A:   Yes! But you should set a definite and measurable task and goal. As in, "I will organize my garage for 20 minutes, minimum, each day. By the end of four weeks the garage must be completely organized."

Q:   As my healthy habit, can I take on more exercise?

A:   You can, but I would encourage you to consider other things. In a recent study of dieters who had lost fifty pounds or more and kept it off, the thing they all had in common was that they had changed things in their life that were unrelated to diet and exercise and therefore seemingly unrelated to weight loss. But as it turns out, keeping an agile mind and an open attitude has a lot to do with maintaining successful weight loss. So—maybe you can take on extra exercise AND something else. E.g.: *For my new healthy habit, I will exercise for an extra 20 minutes a day, and I will journal for 15 minutes.*

Q:   What if an opposing team member picks a lame and easy habit to change? Can I request they pick another habit?

A:   No. You can talk to them about it, but keep in mind that "lame and easy" to you might be cripplingly difficult to your friend. Five minutes of meditation is as hard for me as an hour of ANYTHING ELSE. But when I do it, my mind calms and my spirit improves (and occasionally 5 minutes even morphs into 10). Still, if you think your friend is copping out, talk to her about it. This game is as much about building support and community for a healthy lifestyle as it is about anything else, so it's absolutely fine to ask supportive questions and encourage your teammates to take on more.

## GET A PEN!

On the following lines, write down a few things you think you might like to/need to change. You don't have to officially pick your habits right this second, but writing down the truth will help you narrow down the choices. (And if, after writing, you're still not sure, check out the next chapter, where I've offered some basic instructions on some common healthy habit options.)

_____

_____

_____

_____

_____

_____

_____

_____

_____

_____

_____

_____

## Play by the Rules

- Eliminating an unhealthy habit is worth 10 points per day.
- Integrating a new healthy habit is worth 10 points per day.
- If you change your habits mid-game, you lose 50 points.
- Pick a habit that you want to transform, not something that others think you should change.
- Challenge yourself to think big. The benefit to your life is directly proportional to how big you're willing to go.
- A habit can be anything that affects your physical, emotional, or mental health or quality of life.
- Although we say "think big," you can start small. The important thing is that you begin.
- Old dogs can learn new tricks.

Chapter 13

# HEALTHY HABIT
# INSTRUCTIONS

## (Or, How the Hell Am I Supposed to Do THAT??)

Human beings, who are almost unique
in having the ability to learn from the
experience of others, are also remarkable
for their apparent disinclination to do so.

—*Douglas Noel Adams*

**I'm a big** believer in making things up as I go along. I tend to think that reading too many instruction manuals pulls us away from our instincts and puts us in a mentality of wanting to get a thing right (which usually is the thing that screws us out of having any fun in life—that determination to do it "right"). That said, a little education sometimes goes a really long way. Like, when I was in college and I used the word *penultimate* like this: "The concert was awesome. It was, like, the penultimate entertainment!" I had read the word *penultimate* somewhere and decided it was, like, an even more extreme version of ultimate. My acting professor Rick Seer cocked his head at a funny angle and said, "Um, *penultimate* means second to last. Not super-ultimate." Making it up as I went along had failed me there. Horribly, mortifyingly failed me.

Sometimes we have to learn from people who know. So, like I said in the previous chapter, you can pick almost anything you can think of for your new healthy habit—but if you'd like a little extra guidance, I've included a few of my favorites on the following pages and some basic instructions from people who know much more than I do.

## Yoga

*I was frustrated with how long it took me to get going in the morning (it's like I spent the first couple of hours of my day at half speed) so I took on yoga as my healthy habit. Every morning, first thing after waking, I did a series of Sun Salutations. I can't explain the difference it made in my day. As soon as I completed the series I felt wide awake and raring to go.*

*—Woody, 36*

I love yoga. But I don't do it every day. I have, in my life, gone through phases of doing it every day and when I do, I look better, feel better, and am in general a kinder and funnier person. So why don't I do it every day now? Ummm . . . I don't know. Life gets in the way and somehow my tricky brain convinces me that another cup of coffee will serve me better than putting down my computer and doing a chattaranga or two. I even love that word. Chattaranga. It's basically a push-up, but in yoga, everything sounds prettier.

This latest game, I wanted to restart my yoga practice but I knew I didn't have much time so I simply committed to three Sun Salutations a day. The series takes less than 10 minutes—and stretches just about every muscle in the body, gets your heart rate up, and gets your gratitude flowing. On the following pages are instructions for beginners from my favorite yoga teacher, Jessica Jennings.

• • • • • • • • • • • • • • • • • • • • • • • • • • • • • • • • • • • • •

## The Sun Salutation Series

### Start in Mountain with palms together

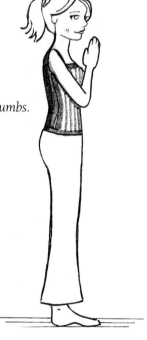

A. *Feet are hips-width and parallel.*
B. *Palms are lightly pressed together with the shoulders drawing back and the chest pressing up toward the thumbs.*
C. *Lift chin slightly to open the throat.*

## Inhale and sweep the arms up, spreading fingers wide

A. *Stay in Mountain alignment with shoulders back*
B. *Look up at the thumbs.*
C. *Lift out of the waist, reaching up toward the sky.*

## Exhale into Forward Fold

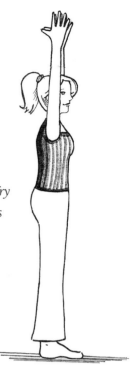

A. *Touch the floor with fingertips, bending the knees if necessary. Try to lift and spread all ten toes to engage the muscles of the legs as you press thighs back toward straight legs.*
B. *Release crown of the head toward the earth.*

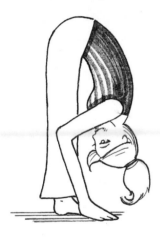

## Inhale and step the right foot back into a Lunge

A. *Make sure the left knee is directly over the ankle.*
B. *Touch the floor on either side of your front foot, melt the upper back down, and lengthen out through crown of the head.*

## Step the left foot back into Plank

A. *The body is one straight line, in a push-up position. Exhale and soften down between the shoulder blades.*

B. *Scoop your tailbone down to draw the belly in and press the heels back.*

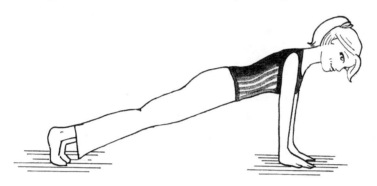

## Exhale down into Four-Limbed Staff Pose

A. *Lower halfway, bending elbows a little away from the body. Keep lifting the shoulders up and back, never lower than the elbows. Bend knees to floor if necessary.*

B. *Breathe.*

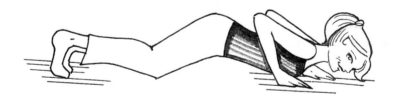

## Inhale into Cobra

A. *Move forward and down to the floor. With bent elbows, pull the shoulders back and pull belly and heart forward. Point nose to the sky.*

B. *Scoop tailbone and lengthen out through your toes.*

C. *Work toward straightening arms as much as you can while keeping head and shoulders back.*

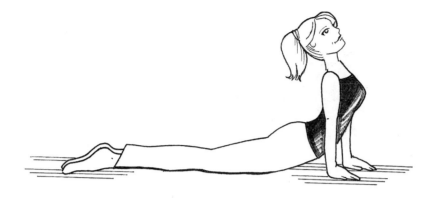

## Exhale into Downward Facing Dog

A. *Tuck the toes under and lift the hips up and back.*

B. *Press fingers firmly down and lift the forearms away from the floor. Soften the upper back down.*

C. *Bend your knees at first to lift the hips and press thighs back to straighten legs. Lift hips up while extending heels down.*

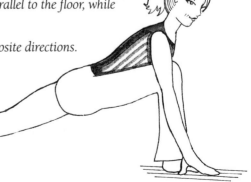

## Inhale and step the right foot forward into a Lunge

A. *Make sure the right knee is directly over the ankle.*

B. *Soften the front thigh down so it's parallel to the floor, while keeping the back thigh lifted.*

C. *Lengthen the bones of the legs in opposite directions.*

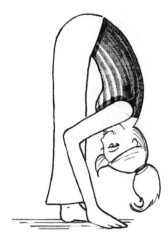

## Exhale and step forward into Forward Fold

A. *Touch the fingertips to the floor, and engage the leg muscles by lifting the kneecaps.*

B. *Press your thighs back toward straight legs.*

C *Lengthen down through crown of head.*

## Inhale and sweep the arms up with palms together

A. *Press the feet down, lift the chest, and look up at the thumbs.*

B. *Root down from tailbone and stretch up and back.*

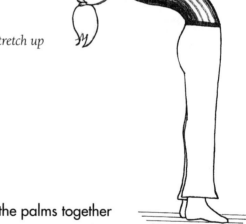

## Exhale and bring the palms together

A. *Come into mountain alignment.*

B. *Palms are lightly pressed together with the shoulders back and the chest broadening into the hands with each breath.*

C. *Root the four corners of the feet down into the earth and stand tall.*

D. *Release the hands to your sides.*

*Ahimsa, the yogic practice of nonviolence, must be adhered to when practicing hatha yoga. Respect your body's limitations and inner wisdom, and if something feels unsafe or painful, please do not do it.*

*Please consult your health care practitioner before starting a yoga practice or any exercise program. Once you decide to proceed, feedback from a trained yoga teacher can make your practice safer and more effective.*

*Jessica Jennings, certified Anusara yoga teacher*
*www.yogagroundwork.com*

• • • • • • • • • • • • • • • • • • • • • • • • • • • • • • • • •

Personally, I LOVE the Sun Salutation series. And it's really not hard to learn. But if it feels like too much for you to begin with, then consider these instructions on how to do yoga ANYWHERE from Jennifer Bloom. If you take this on as your healthy habit, then you might commit to something like this: *I will not make phone calls in the car. Or, I will not stand around hating smelly people on the subway. Instead, I will practice yoga.* And then do it every day, every drive, or every ride and see what happens to your mood and your life!

• • • • • • • • • • • • • • • • • • • • • • • • • • • • • • • • • • • • • • • • • • • • • •

## Yoga Anywhere

• • • • • • • • • • • • • • • • • • • • • • • • • • • • • • • • • • • • • • • • • • • • • •

If you're considering checking out yoga, believe me, it's one of the coolest things you can do for yourself. EVERYTHING changes—not just the size and shape of your body, but your self-esteem, your mood, your creativity, your sex life, your ability to love and be passionate, compassionate, patient . . . all those things we know instinctively we'd like to cultivate but aren't really sure how to start and don't really have the time for.

I'm a guerilla yogini. Yes, I teach in studios and classrooms, but I also find ways for the rest of the world to fold it into busy lives.

Here are a few guidelines to building a yoga practice for the car, on the phone, or anywhere else you find yourself stuck:

**Breath:** Establish a slow, steady breath pattern. Inhale for a slow count of 5. Hold full for a count of 1, then exhale for a count of 6, just a touch longer than your inhale. Every exhale produces a metabolic change as you release carbon dioxide and cell debris and is another chance to get rid of tension, stale air, and stale thoughts.

**Circles:** Now that you have a slow, steady breath, try making circles. Our body is full of circles—you can circle the head, the shoulders, the ribs, wrists, ankles, even the tailbone! (That's my favorite, like belly dancing in the car.) Try doing half a circle on the inhale, and half the circle on the exhale. Or circle in one direction as you breathe in, the other direction as you breathe out. You can work through the spine and body sequentially in this manner—doing several sets for each body part, almost like a corkscrew.

**Open Heart:** Practice your compassion by opening your heart. At each stoplight, take a hand off the steering wheel (just one, please), and place it directly over your head on the ceiling of the car. Now, walk your hand toward the back windshield. You should feel a tremendous stretch through the armpit and into the muscles of the chest. Hold here for several slow, deep breaths. Play with the position of your hand, maybe reaching further toward either of the back corners of the car—make this stretch perfect for you. As you peel away the tension around your heart, you may be able to find a bit more freedom to love yourself and the other drivers sharing the road with you.

Bottom line is, ANY yoga is better than no yoga. I'm a cancer survivor. Already a yogini when diagnosed, I practiced this introspective, subtler, guerilla yoga at the doctor's office, in the chemo chair, on the phone with the insurance people—everywhere! It saved me a lot of tears and drama and helped get me to complete remission in six months.

The coolest thing about yoga? You'll shed weight, anxiety, and boredom in buckets. You'll end up doing things physically, mentally, cre-atively, and emotionally that you never thought you'd be able to do. And you're helping to achieve world peace, by starting with yourself.

*Jennifer Bloom, RYT, is the creative director of Yogablooms. She conducts workshops on Guerilla Yoga and Yoga and Cancer, and regularly teaches yoga to all ages and sizes in Los Angeles, www.yogablooms.com*

• • • • • • • • • • • • • • • • • • • • • • • • • • • • • • •

# Journaling

*At first I thought I had nothing to write about. And then after a couple of days, I had everything to write about! It felt so good to spill the ugly truth—the craziness and fears and pettiness and silliness that goes through my mind—even just to myself and my journal.*

—Leah, 30

In a slew of studies, journaling has been shown to radically decrease stress, radically improve mood, and even improve physical health. So how do you do it? You do it by knowing that you can't do it wrong! Put pen to paper. But maybe knowing this little stat will help: *Researchers have found that people who write about their deepest thoughts and feelings surrounding upsetting events have stronger immunity and visit their doctors half as often as those who write only about trivial events.* Crazy, huh? That the act of putting pen to paper and spilling your feelings on to the page can actually reduce your stress enough to improve your immune system??

That statistic actually doesn't surprise me that much because I am absolutely convinced that the act of journaling is the main thing that kept me sane through my pretty chaotic childhood, teens, and twenties. I was an obsessive journal writer from the age of eight when my mom gave my sister Kaili and me these pretty, shiny Asian-style journals for Christmas. I didn't know what to write in mine so I snuck and read Kaili's and then COPIED the first few sentences she'd written! True story. Which I think she is just now learning for the first time.

Hee. It went something like this (I know—'cause I still have it). "Dear Diary, I think diary is not a good name for you. I love you! So I think I will name you Love. Yeah, that's a good name! Dear Love . . ." Hee. Hee Hee. I kept journals from the age of eight until the age of twenty-eight and then stopped abruptly. And in writing this chapter, I sat in my fluffy green chair for a long time trying to figure WHY I stopped. I have boxes and boxes of journals—through grade school, high school, and college, through my New York waitressing years, my Portland acting years, and my early years in L.A. when I was trying desperately to get an agent. And then they just *stop*. I couldn't figure it out for a while, so I went back and read the last few I have.

And then it came to me. I stopped journaling when I got a good therapist, which tells me for certain that my journals served as therapist to me for a long, long time. They are full of pain, full of heartbreak, full of bad poetry. There is not a lot of happiness in them—I tended to stop writing during my happiest times, and then start again when life fell apart. There is no doubt that they were my best friend, my secret keeper, my dumping ground, and that they held my sanity in their well worn pages . . . *Dear Diary, I think diary is not a good name for you. So I think I will name you Love. Yeah, that's a good name. Dear Love . . . That Kaili. Pretty wise for a ten-year-old.*

If you're tempted to try but are not sure where to start, let's look at a couple of techniques from some of my favorite teachers.

In her bestselling book *The Artist's Way,* Julia Cameron encourages the act of "unconscious writing." She suggests putting pen to paper and writing, ceaselessly and without pause for thought, until you've filled up three pages. This way you're taking your editing eye, your desire to be "correct," out of it and just letting your unconscious be your guide. She calls them "morning pages" and suggests you do your writing first thing in the morning—in order to get all the blather out of your head and onto the page before you start your day.

In her wonderful book *Writing Down the Bones,* Natalie Goldberg suggests a similar kind of automatic writing. She suggests you set a timer for 10 or 15 minutes and then start writing and keep your pen moving till the timer goes off. Don't stop to correct spelling mistakes or punctuation. Just write. And if you run out of things to write, write that. So it might look something like this: *I don't want to go to work today, my boss is mad at her boss and I don't like her boss either and I think that guy who sits across from me in that cubicle is really cute and I don't know what to wear also I'm scared of terrorists and I don't know what to write, I'm out of things. Can't think of anything else oh yeah, my dad is driving me craaaazy with his craziness. I'm worried he might die soon.* It doesn't have to track. It doesn't have to make sense to anyone but you. It doesn't even have to make sense to you. The pen just has to keep moving.

You can do it in the morning like Julia Cameron suggests or you can do it at night—which can be a great way to improve your night's sleep. Get all the blather from the day out of your head and onto the page—putting it to rest so that you can put yourself to rest! Either way, put pen to paper and let your hand go. Let it be nonsensical. Let it be emotional. Let it be annoying or crazy. Let it be whatever it wants to be. Just write. Try it right now! Fill up these blank lines and see if you don't just feel a little better! (And if you do, commit to it for the next twenty-eight days!)

---------------------------------------------------------------

---------------------------------------------------------------

---------------------------------------------------------------

---------------------------------------------------------------

---------------------------------------------------------------

---------------------------------------------------------------

---------------------------------------------------------------

---------------------------------------------------------------

---------------------------------------------------------------

---------------------------------------------------------------

---------------------------------------------------------------

---------------------------------------------------------------

---------------------------------------------------------------

---------------------------------------------------------------

---------------------------------------------------------------

---------------------------------------------------------------

---------------------------------------------------------------

# Meditation

*The game got me to meditate. For real. Every day. A simple thing,
right? Not for me. Even though meditation shifts my entire day, makes
me feel better, helps keep me calm and centered and focused, I was
never willing to do it on a regular basis—until I made it my good habit
in the game. Then I had to do it—or risk letting down my team. And
once I got in the habit, it stuck with me. I've meditated (almost) every
day, ever since—even when I'm not playing the game. That may not
sound like a big deal, but if you were my yoga teacher you'd understand how freaking amazing that is.*

*—Peter, 39*

For me, personally, nothing is harder than forcing myself to sit down
and meditate. Sitting still is excruciating for me. Watching my thoughts
skitter through my chaotic mind is excruciating for me. Letting those
thoughts go—without judgment—is next to impossible for me. But the
best advice I ever got on this came from my yoga teacher Jessica Jennings
when I said, "I hate meditating. All I do is sit around and think about how
mad I am at my husband and how worried I am about what's going on at
work." And she said, "Yeah, but after meditating, at least you know that. At
least you noticed. If you hadn't meditated, you might just sit around eating
mindlessly or feeling anxious all day and have no idea why." Hmmmm . . .
interesting.

But I still hate it. So why, when I actually do it, even for 5 minutes, do
I feel so damn good after? I am here to attest that despite my every instinct
screaming at me not to bother, when I do bother, I *always* find meditation
calming at a level I find difficult to describe. (But I'll try.) When I was a
kid, my mom would take me to visit my godmother, Berta, who married
a Navajo medicine man and lived on the Navajo reservation. When we
would stay with Berta, and I would be scared to fall asleep because maybe
I'd just seen a weird-looking lizard or snake skittering around outside,
Berta would lie down beside me and rub my temples, really gently and
lovingly, until I would fall asleep. It's like the feel of her fingers calmed all

of my nerves and soothed all of my fears, made me feel safe, made me feel protected, helped me know I wasn't alone.

Meditation, as hard as it can be, ultimately feels like that, like a loving godmother's fingers on the temples of a frightened child. So that's my pitch.

If you're in, or think you might be in, here are some instructions just for us by meditation teacher Michael Bernard Beckwith, founder of the Agape International Spiritual Center and author of *Spiritual Liberation: Fulfilling Your Soul's Potential.*

• • • • • • • • • • • • • • • • • • • • • • • • • • • • • • • • • • • • • • • • • •

## Meditation for Beginners

• • • • • • • • • • • • • • • • • • • • • • • • • • • • • • • • • • • • • • • • • •

There are many motivations for meditating. Some individuals have read the results of the many medical studies that report the health benefits of meditation, such as slowing down one's heart rate and reducing stress levels. Others may become interested for psychological purposes including self-observation, insights into habitual patterns, and so on. Then there are spiritual motives such as deepening one's intuition, mindfulness, or enlightenment, which is spiritual liberation.

In the meditation classes and retreats I conduct, I invite individuals to first understand their motive for embarking on a meditative journey. Your motive may include a combination of purposes just described, or something entirely different. The good news is that once you begin to taste the sweet fruits of meditating, you will realize that there is no aspect of your life that is not affected.

You may begin by selecting a space conducive to gathering your energies and centering yourself. You needn't devote an entire room or construct an elaborate shrine or altar, but assigning a specific location will have an accumulative affect and "build" the energy of meditation. Then, on days when sitting is challenging, the energy of your meditation spot will assist you.

Plan to allow for about 10 to 20 minutes if you are a beginning practitioner. And don't be surprised if it feels just short of eternity! At first it is startling to observe the contents of your mind—the speediness, busyness, and restlessness, especially if you have never witnessed your thought processes. There is a natural urge to find justifiable reasons for leaping from your cushion or chair. This is where a sense of humor enters in. There is no thought—whether it's about work, sex, food, your mother-in-law—that is unacceptable. These are just the things that roll through. Observe them just as you do a cloud that is passing through the sky.

Sit on a firm chair with a straight back. Sit away from the back of the chair with your feet flat on the floor and your palms resting on your thighs in the downward or upward position. You may either close your eyes or, leaving them open, gently cast your glance downward about six feet in front of you. If you are sitting on a floor cushion, whether you sit cross-legged or not, use a second pillow so that your hips are higher than your knees so that your back is properly supported. If you feel guided to begin with a prayer or affirmative statement, do so.

Slowly begin to center yourself by becoming aware of your inhalations and exhalations, without regulating your breath. Just breathe naturally. At first you may become self-conscious of your breath, causing you to attempt to control it, but in time this will stop. Begin to contemplate your oneness with life's Source, or with all Existence, whatever that may mean to you. Consider that you are not alone as you meditate, that you are being held, uplifted, and supported by all the other individuals who are in the meditative field of awareness.

Once you are centered, with each exhalation notice that there is an accompanying gap, where only your breath is taking place. If your mind has wandered, simply bring yourself back to center by saying, "thinking." Don't be frustrated by the discursiveness of your thoughts, which are common to all meditators no matter how much mileage they have! Consider your thoughts like a cloud in the sky, just floating by, which is what will help you not to get hooked and carried away with them.

At the end of your meditation period, you may close with a prayer or affirmative thought and set an intention to be mindful throughout your day. Little by little, you will become aware of so many things to be grateful for, like the beauty of nature and your growing sense of interconnectedness to others and all life.

As you deepen your interiority through meditation, you will become acquainted with yourself and your Authentic Self in a magnificent way. Do not underestimate the simplicity of this Vipassana technique. The results at first are subtle, but will become profoundly influential in your life. You may supplement your meditation by exploring the writings of meditation teachers or spiritual organizations that conduct meditation sessions in your town.

*Michael Berrard Beckwith, founder of the Agape*
*International Spiritual Center, author*

. . . . . . . . . . . . . . . . . . . . . . . . . . . . . .

Meditation may seem a little woo woo to you at first, or really difficult or scary or nonsensical. But keep this in mind: In a recent study, Dr. Inga Treitler, Ph.D., a cultural anthropologist, studied a group of people who successfully lost a lot of weight and kept it off and she found that they all had one thing in common:

"All the subjects had incorporated some meditative element into their lives," Treitler says. "It might have been walking or yoga, but it was self time, a white space where they could disengage from the old, obsessive behavior."

So try it. Sit down. Sit still. Breathe. You might hate it. Or it might completely transform your life.

# Decluttering Your Life

*The healthy habit I took on was to organize and clear clutter for half an hour each day. It improved my life because my house looks pretty and my husband isn't irritated by all the clutter! I also put away my clothes every day—no piles on the hamper—and I've managed to keep that going—not perfectly, but better than before.*

*—Kate, 37*

You know that movie *The Secret*? How you can manifest a new reality by, like, thinking about it? My including this section in this book is maybe my first attempt at manifesting some decluttering in my life. I have, at this moment, 15,324 e-mails in my in-box. Of those, 634 are unread. They date back to 1999. I shit you not. And this? This is indicative of how I function in every other aspect of my life. I have paperwork everywhere that I don't need. Books piled everywhere that I've never read. If I didn't have an assistant who has made it her personal daily goal to file every piece of paper I scatter . . . ? Her name is Star, by the way, and I'm convinced that's because she was literally dropped from the starry heavens into my life because I *cannot survive* without her. Seriously, you'd find me dead, buried under a pile of scripts, take-out containers, and empty coffee cups. Point is that I do not have the foggiest idea how one would begin to declutter—but I have tracked down someone who does: Fay Wolf, organizing expert. Let's all listen, shall we?

• • • • • • • • • • • • • • • • • • • • • • • • • • • • • • • • • • • • • • • • • • •
## Getting Organized
• • • • • • • • • • • • • • • • • • • • • • • • • • • • • • • • • • • • • • • • • • •

*Use it, love it, or leave it.* That's the first thing you need to know about clearing your space and mind. Burn that mantra into your noggin and you are halfway there. The second golden nugget? *Small steps.* Got 30 minutes or less per day? Perfect. Just because something might take longer than 30 minutes to *finish* doesn't mean you can't work on it for 30 minutes and then stop. *Some done* is better than *none done*. And indeed, many organizing tasks take only 30 minutes or less, from start to finish. Try these small steps to keep clutter at bay.

**Mail:** Personally, I've always loved getting the mail. Most folks, on the other hand, dread the continuous flow of what is, these days, mostly junk. But snuck in between all the stuff we never asked for is the stuff we actually need to deal with. (And sometimes? *Money.* As a professional organizer, I have found a total of more than $15,000 in undeposited checks in clients' homes!) As soon as the mail comes in the door, open it, unfold it, recycle the envelopes and the filler that comes with bills, and place the keepers in a specified in-box (*one* area designated for incoming paper). You don't have to take action on your mail every day. You just have to *open it.* It'll take 5 to 10 minutes per day, *tops.*

**Piles of paper:** Take a stack of paper from your in-box (or from one of those many piles that litter the once-gorgeous home you pay all that money to live in), and take thirty minutes to sort. Most paper falls into one of three categories: TO DO, TO FILE, TOSS. Don't worry about actually doing or filing anything . . . *yet.* Break it down. Sort it out. Move on. (The final steps with paper will be making appointments with yourself to take action and file those papers. *Keep those appointments.*)

**Get rid of it:** Create a donation area near the entryway. Perhaps a basket that stays there year-round. There is ALWAYS stuff to purge. Life changes, needs change, fashions change. Ask yourself: Can I live happily without this item? Nine times out of ten, the answer is YES. Even 15 minutes in your clothes closet could yield a few garbage bags' worth of stuff that you forgot you had, no longer fits, has holes or stains, or belonged to an ex who's long gone. When the donation area is full, fill up some bags to go to charity. And then *bring it there.* (Or, in most states, you can call the Salvation Army or Vietnam Veterans of America and they will come pick it up!)

**Make a deal—and stick to it:** Bargain with yourself. You'll spend 20 to 30 minutes on a quick organizing task, and THEN you get to watch *Grey's Anatomy.* Parent yourself a little bit. And also *reward yourself.* Living a life of clarity takes a little work. But man, oh, man, is it worth it. Happy organizing!

—*Fay Wolf, organizing expert and owner of*
*NEW ORDER Professional Organizing, www.neworderorganizing.com*

• • • • • • • • • • • • • • • • • • • • • • • • • • • •

# Learn or Practice a Musical Instrument

*The game inspired me to finally learn to play the piano in my living room. I sounded like a kid at the keys in the beginning, driving my wife and neighbors crazy with the scales. But for some reason, the whole thing just filled me with glee. I can now play the theme to Indiana Jones—with both hands! Awesome.*

—Kevin, 42

I am a music junkie. I love to sing and I love to write songs. I spent my late teens and early twenties dating men who played the guitar, and writing songs with them. Then when we would break up, they always got custody of the songs because I couldn't play the guitar. So one of my first conscious acts of feminism was to put an end to that. I spent one diligent summer learning to play. Now, no one would call me a guitar player. I do not play artfully. I do not play well. But I play well enough to write songs (which really requires only about three chords).

When I play and sing, it fills my soul up and takes away my worries and is its own kind of meditation for me—but when my life gets busy, the first thing that falls away is the guitar. So in my very first game, the healthy habit I took on was to practice my guitar 20 minutes a day. I was amazed what I could accomplish in only 20 minutes! And it's not just me, and it's not because I already could play a little. My friend Mandy has a job, twin three-year-old boys, and a four-month-old daughter, and she just challenged herself to learn to play guitar. I promise you she's lucky if she finds anywhere *near* 20 minutes a day—and yet, after only about a month, she has learned several chords and a tricky little scale that I can't even do!

Here's what else: Researchers have found that music-making is not only fun, it not only decreases stress, it not only provides a boost in self-esteem, it also improves the mind, increases mental clarity, and may help to ward off Alzheimer's disease and other dementias. One study found that people who took keyboard lessons showed decreases in anxiety, depression, and loneliness, and significantly increased levels of human growth hormone.

Another found that patients with Alzheimer's disease who underwent four weeks of structured music therapy showed significant increases in their level of melatonin, a neurohormone linked with sleep regulation and believed to influence the immune system. So how much do you have to practice to get all these benefits? *Not that much at all.*

If you can afford to, buy an instrument. Buy the one you really want to play. Buy it used, buy it at a thrift store, buy the cheapest one you can find. And if you can't afford to buy, you can rent one really inexpensively. Consider how much money you've spent on things like a visit to the doctor to deal with depression or sleeplessness, and the cost actually feels quite low! Then, either hire a teacher and take a class once a week, buy a lesson on DVD, or download free lessons/instructions from the Internet. Come on. You know you've always wanted to learn. And no one's gonna do it for you. The time is now! Take it on and then let's have a sing-along! (And now, a word from an actual music teacher.)

• • • • • • • • • • • • • • • • • • • • • • • • • • • • • • • • • • • • • • • • • •
## Music for Beginners
• • • • • • • • • • • • • • • • • • • • • • • • • • • • • • • • • • • • • • • • • •

Often, we try to take on too much, get frustrated with the lack of progress, and quit before we feel our success. The key is to create little bite-size successes.

Here are some pointers to get started with learning music and make it fun!

### Listen:

Music is in all of us, and half of learning music is in the listening. So start with 20 minutes of focused listening every day. Find some of your favorite songs, sit back, close your eyes, and listen. Listen in a way that you have never listened before. In your mind, start separating the various parts that make up the song. Piano, guitar, rhythm, vocals, etc.

### Stick with the basics:

Everything is made up of small components, just like atoms make up matter. Start recognizing the basic roots of music: notes and chords. Take guitar for example. Start by learning one basic chord, and slowly become comfortable playing it. Do this by yourself using online tools or with a teacher. Have fun! There is nothing to lose! Now, try learning a second chord. Slowly practice going back and forth between the two chords. It will seem impossible . . . until it becomes easy . . . and then it becomes second nature.

### Songs:

Think of one of your favorite songs, and find the chords online. (Find one that has only a few, relatively easy chords.) Then learn those chords and practice the song for 20 minutes a day. This is the process of little bite-size successes, because now you are playing something that you love, and that is the most important thing!

*Deepak Ramapriyan*
*www.theotherdeepak.com*

•  •  •  •  •  •  •  •  •  •  •  •  •  •  •  •  •  •  •  •  •  •  •  •  •

# Study a Foreign Language

*I always wanted to learn to speak Spanish but figured I didn't have the money for a class or the time to study. But with the Internet, you can learn for free and half an hour a day is about all the studying my brain can take anyway. I'm not fluent yet—but I'm determined to get there!*
*—Andie, 33*

In the eighth grade, I failed French 1. Class was at eight in the morning, for God's sake! I sooo preferred sleeping in to showing up to Miss Sasso's class to learn how to conjugate a verb. Shoulda gone, though, 'cause I just had to take it again the next year. I took four (or, if you count the repeat, five) years of high school French. I did not excel, but I got by. I would have told you I hadn't retained any of it, except that when I was twenty-two I got to go backpacking through Bolivia and Peru for a month. I spent the weeks prior and the plane ride over poring through English to Spanish dictionaries. And when I finally arrived in Cuzco, I opened my mouth to speak Spanish . . . and the only thing that came out was French.

For weeks, I mortified myself and my friends by meaning to say *por favor* and managing only a sheepish *s'il vous plaît*. Then, finally, the Spanish kicked in. And, of course, when I finally got to go to Paris years later—I could only remember Spanish. I don't speak either language very well, but Miss Sasso's class gave me a foundation for which I am grateful. And I'm especially grateful for it now that I've read about all the mental benefits to be gained from learning a foreign language.

Believe it or not, studies have shown that learning a foreign language can literally create gray matter in your brain! They show too that learning a foreign language is a FANTASTIC deterrent to the effects of aging on the brain. By learning a language, you are actually benefiting your health and your mood as well as the world by saying, hey, most of y'all don't speak English (more than four-fifths of the world's inhabitants don't speak English) so I'm willing to step outside myself and my upbringing and try to meet you halfway! If you need some added inspiration, read *Eat, Pray, Love*, by Elizabeth Gilbert. I promise you won't get through fifty pages before you're convinced that you must learn Italian for the sheer sexiness of it!

But for some actual instructions, let's listen to Laurie Ferguson (no relation to Az), a language specialist who's been teaching English as a second language both in the States and abroad for many years.

• • • • • • • • • • • • • • • • • • • • • • • • • • • • • • • • • • • • • • • • •
## Learning a New Language
• • • • • • • • • • • • • • • • • • • • • • • • • • • • • • • • • • • • • • • • •

If you want to study a foreign language start by choosing a language you'd *love* to learn. Don't study it because you ought to; study it because you'd love to. Next, go to your library or go online and choose a language learning kit that includes a book and a comprehensive audio component (cassettes, CDs, MP3 downloads—whatever works for your lifestyle). Then, use the learning kit to get started, but don't be a slave to it. Try to spend time with it every day and remember that a little time every day is much more useful than sporadic, long study stretches. Especially when it comes to studying vocabulary . . . less time and more frequency is much more effective (and fun) than marathon drilling sessions.

Your learning kit will most likely present vocabulary groups but if there are words or groups of words that are important to you in your own life pull out your dictionary and, by all means, learn your favorite words first. Keep vocabulary learning fun and interesting; learn active verbs by acting them out while saying them. Label every object in your kitchen with a sticky note, listen to your vocab words and their translations while taking a walk, download software with a vocabulary screensaver ("virtual teacher software"), or listen to vocab words and their translations in the car, on the treadmill, while folding laundry, etc. Be creative!

Also, learn lots of common words and cognates. By learning the most commonly used 100 words in a language (such as *the, and, but)* you get a lot of bang for your vocabulary buck. Cognates (words that are very similar in English and the new language) are freebies. They are quick to learn and accumulate in your memory quickly.

Next, find opportunities to hear and read the target language in the real world. Buy a foreign language newspaper, tune in to a foreign language radio station or TV station or Web film, or rent a foreign language film. Find lots of opportunities to see and hear the language being used in contexts that interest you.

Don't get too hung up on grammar in the beginning stages. Learn what you can from the program you've chosen and remember that there'll be plenty of time to worry about grammar later and only very basic grammar is needed to achieve basic communication.

Next, find yourself a language partner. Meet with a native speaker of your target language who would like the opportunity to practice conversational English. Get together for coffee and chat it up—first in one language and then in the other. There are English learners all over the country who want a chance to practice English in the company of a native speaker. There are ads for language partners all over college campuses, international centers, newspapers, etc.

The most important thing is to always remember that the whole purpose of language is communication. That is important to keep in mind so that as you progress with the process you don't get hung up on speaking perfectly. Keep the focus on understanding and being understood. Many second language learners are hesitant to talk in the target language because they are afraid to make mistakes. Let that go and realize that the important thing is just getting your point across.

*Laurie Sansone Ferguson, language and literacy specialist*

• • • • • • • • • • • • • • • • • • • • • • • • • • • • • • • • •

# Be of Loving Service to Others

*My girlfriend Fran and I created a group called the Guerrilla Givers. Badass givers who perform random acts of kindness around L.A. Two of our outings were handing out flowers on Valentine's Day and giving free hugs on the Third Street promenade. EVERYONE should try it!*
*—Duffy, 39*

This is my favorite section of this whole book because I actually think it's the key to life and love and happiness. When I was getting sober in my twenties and suffering all the narcissistic agony that comes with getting sober in your twenties, I was given this piece of advice: "When you feel like crap, find someone who feels worse than you and offer to help them out." Single best piece of advice I've ever been given. Second to that was, "When you're resenting the hell out of somebody, pray for them and then show them an act of kindness." The wise friends who told me to do this called it "taking contrary action."

When I want to kill my boss because she hasn't noticed how hard I've been working, I take a breath and then observe, to her, out loud, how hard *she's* been working. I don't do it bitterly. I don't do it so she'll do it in kind. I do it because she is working incredibly hard. And it's how hard she's working that has prevented her from noticing how hard I'm working. And complimenting her gets me out of my selfishness and neediness, and I feel better. And suddenly I don't need her to return the favor (though quite often she does).

If I'm at the grocery store and the clerk is moving really slowly and my inclination is to throttle him, I smile at him instead. Usually, he's moving slowly because he's panicked and overwhelmed and sees that everybody is mad at him and a simple smile from a stranger is what he needs to calm down and do his job better. And even if it isn't, smiling is what I need to calm down and live my life better. I am not a saint. I do not practice this perfectly. But when I do practice it? Everything—absolutely everything—feels better. (My favorite story about this very thing is in Anne Lamott's brilliant book *Plan B*. The story is called "Ham of God" and if you haven't read it, you truly must.)

And by the way? This isn't just my hippie dippie theory. Many studies have been conducted on the powers of kindness, and studies repeatedly find that the feeling of well-being that comes from helping and showing kindness to others has very real psychological and physical benefits. It improves your self-worth, improves your mood, alleviates anxiety and depression, and releases natural endorphins, which reduce both stress and physical pain. Don't believe it? Awesome! Be your own scientist; test the theory!

So how do you quantify it for the game? Well, you could go to www .volunteermatch.org and ask them to pair you up with a charity in your neighborhood that you can work for a little every day. Or you can choose from this list of small ideas for kindness, and you can do one every day, or you can take on one big project (like a charity drive) and work on it for half an hour each day. And then watch how your whole life (or at least your whole mood) *transforms*.

## Ideas For Kindness

### Volunteer to be a tutor in a school or at a local library
Read to children or teach illiterate adults to read.

### Donate time at a senior center
You can cook, you can sing, you can bring your baby for a visit. It will raise their spirits and yours!

## Give blood

Better yet, organize a group of friends to come give blood with you. People need it every day and most of us go only in the wake of a crisis.

## Organize a neighborhood clean up

If that's too much for you, just commit to pick up litter wherever you see it.

## Drop off fresh flowers or fresh baked treats to your local police or fire department

Add a personalized thank-you note for all they do.

## Write or call an old teacher and tell him or her what she meant to you

If you can afford it, enclose some money, tell them you're sorry that teachers are so woefully underpaid, and that dinner tonight is on you.

## Give a bag of groceries, a take-out meal, or a homemade sandwich to a homeless person

Or, if you have more time than money, volunteer at a local shelter or soup kitchen. They need help every day, and most of us think to volunteer only on holidays.

## Wash a car, mow a lawn, rake leaves, or shovel snow for an elderly neighbor

Or, if you're a mom, offer to babysit for another neighborhood mom free of charge.

## Help animals in need

If you're an animal lover, collect food, toys, kitty litter, towels, and soft blankets and donate them—as well as any extra time you have—to your local animal shelter.

## A Few More Ideas for Your New Healthy Habit

**Call three people you like each day.** Remember when we used to actually talk to each other? If you're in your twenties or younger, then maybe you don't. But back in the day? Before e-mailing and texting and IMing and Facebook? We used to actually pick up this old-fashioned thing called a telephone or, and this is radical, go see a neighbor *in person* and sit and chat over a cup of tea. We are so easily connected these days and yet so completely disconnected. How many times have you had a misunderstanding with a friend because you misinterpreted their intended tone in an e-mail? So commit to reaching out to three people a day with your actual voice and see if you don't end up feeling a whole lot better.

**Cook a meal at home every day and eat it at the dinner table.** The act of cooking can be both social and enjoyable. This is a fantastic way to reconnect with yourself and your loved ones. It's supereasy to get buried in work and technology and take-out containers and completely lose touch with the person who sleeps in the bed next to you or the bedroom next to yours. Turn off the TV and the computer and turn on the stove. It doesn't have to be elaborate. Scramble some egg whites and veggies and chop up a salad and talk to each other while you do it. If you want to get really wild, wash the dishes together after you eat. Now that's just craaaazy!

**Read.**

**Floss.**

**Or read and floss.** Because flossing takes only a couple of minutes and I think you can manage a little bit more.

Okay. That's it for the instructions. I'm not gonna teach you how to floss your teeth or read. (Though reading is a very popular choice in the game. It's amazing how many of us haven't read a good book in years!) Okay, fine, I'm not gonna teach you how to read but I will tell you some of my favorite books, just to give you a little kick-start in that direction. In no particular order . . .

*Traveling Mercies* by Anne Lamott. My favorite book maybe ever.

*The Handmaid's Tale* by Margaret Atwood. My favorite book when I was in high school, recommended by my wonderful English teacher Linda Fowler.

*Another Roadside Attraction* by Tom Robbins. My favorite book when I was in college, with some of the best sex scenes ever.

*One Hundred Years of Solitude* by Gabriel García Márquez. Pure magic. My favorite book from my twenties. Best read while backpacking through South America.

*A Heartbreaking Work of Staggering Genius* by Dave Eggers. Appropriately titled. My favorite book after my dad died. It made me feel less alone.

*The Glass Castle* by Jeannette Walls. Made me grateful for every moment of my life. My favorite book in recent years.

*Bee Season* by Myla Goldberg. Blew my mind. Just read it. Seriously. Right now.

*The Corrections* by Jonathan Franzen. Reading it made me a better writer.

## • • • A Tip from Az • • •

I don't really have a tip for you here. Just some of my favorite books.

*The Seven Spiritual Laws of Success* by Deepak Chopra. Fundamentally changed the way I look at the world.

*The Master Key System* by Charles Haanel. All about meditation and manifestation—and the author encourages you to read only one chapter per week. Marvelous.

*To Kill a Mockingbird* by Harper Lee. Read this when I was about eight and have continued to read it every couple of years since.

*True and False* by David Mamet. Read this just after leaving school, and wish I had read it before.

*The Tibetan Book of Living and Dying* by Sogyal Rinpoche. Opened up my perspective on life.

*Oh, the Places You'll Go!* by Dr. Seuss. I love this book. And it's profound, even when I read it now.

# GET A PEN!

List your favorite books and what you love about them . . . Then trade lists with a teammate!

_____
_____
_____
_____
_____
_____
_____
_____
_____
_____
_____
_____
_____
_____
_____
_____
_____
_____
_____

• • • • • • • • • • • • • • • • • • • • • • • • • • • • • • • • • •
### Step Up Your Game!
• • • • • • • • • • • • • • • • • • • • • • • • • • • • • • • • • •

Form a mini book club with your team! You can all commit to reading for half an hour a night and then you can go for long, speedy walks together and talk about the book.

Okay, I'm really done now. I'm really, really not gonna teach you how to floss.

Crap. Fine. I will.

## How to Floss

1. Pull a foot or two of floss from the floss container. Wrap it around the pointer fingers of both hands and pull it taut.
2. Slip floss between your teeth and into the area between your teeth and gums as far as it will go without you drooling blood. (Though if you're not a flosser, you actually may bleed a little the first few times because your gums will be sensitive.)
3. Floss with several strokes to dislodge food and plaque.
4. Do all your teeth at least once every day.
5. You can floss before or after you brush your teeth. The most important time to floss is before bedtime. If you get sleepy and lazy right before bed, consider flossing while you watch TV after dinner.
6. SMILE FOR YOUR DENTIST. She will be so very proud!

Okay, for reals. That's it. The end. Bye, now. Turn the page. Oh! Wait! Before you turn the page . . .

## GET A PEN!

Write down a few ideas of what your new healthy habit might be! You can choose from this chapter or make up some of your own.

_____

_____

_____

_____

_____

_____

_____
_____
_____
_____
_____
_____
_____
_____
_____
_____
_____
_____
_____
_____
_____

Jo O'Key, *15 pounds lost*

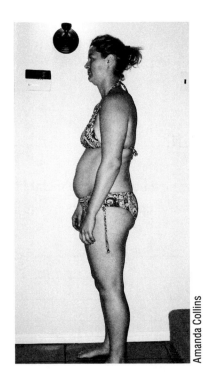
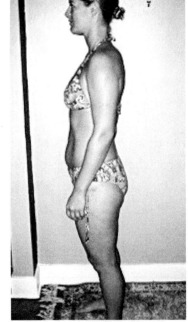

Amanda Collins

I took on the game because of my ever-expanding ass and my ever-increasing discomfort with the size of it. I'm highly competitive in everything I do — and I actually kicked off my weight loss by secretly (like, I knew it, but they didn't) competing with some girlfriends who were trying to lose weight too! But the game took it to the next level, allowing me to pull my competitive instincts out of hiding and revel in the fact that it now felt like a big team sport!

The camaraderie was awesome. We shared recipes and also upsets all along the way. Mood swings, victories, disappointments, and excitement in results. Yet all the way we maintained this great attitude of "I'll help you and wish you do well for your body and all that but I am secretly going to do better than you so there!" And I loved that.

The game rocks! I'm doing it again this month so look out. I'll kick your big, fat butt! By the way, I lost most of mine.

JoJo, 33

Chapter 14

# ALCOHOL, COFFEE, AND DIET SODA

### (Or, What Do You Mean I Can't Drink All My Calories?)

One reason I don't drink is that
I want to know when I'm having a good time.

—*Nancy Astor*

# Alcohol

**The Rules:** No alcohol is to be consumed while you are playing the game except on the day off. You may also have one portion during the meal off.

**The Penalty:** If you consume alcohol at unsanctioned times, you lose *25 points per portion*. A portion is up to 12 ounces of beer, 6 ounces of wine, or 1.5 ounces of hard liquor.

**The Escalation:** If you don't make weight on any given week, you lose the privilege of alcohol on your day off *for the duration of the game*.

**The truth is,** this rule wasn't really a difficult thing for me because I haven't had a drink since I was twenty-two. It's not that I don't like drinking; it's that I like it a little too much. It's also that when I drink I become desperate and needy and sloppy and start fistfights in bars with people who are much bigger and maler than I am. Also, I watched alcohol destroy too many people I love, so I made a decision pretty early in life to not be one of them. Quitting drinking at twenty-two was not easy. But with help from some wonderful, like-minded souls, I did it. It makes me *incredibly happy* that my daughter will never see me drunk and that in making that one subversive, radical decision, I have averted and rewritten a toxic family cycle that went back for many generations . . . Duuuuuude. I just got all serious on you. Heh. I like to change it up sometimes. Keep you guessing.

Okay, so this rule wasn't a thing for me, but my friend Richard? HATED it. He was all excited to play the game and lose the pudge around the middle, but the idea of giving up his nightly beer? Heeeelllll, no. He was all, "I work hard, dammit! I WORK REALLY HARD. Long, LONG hours of work. I *earn* my beer. I *deserve* my beer. I *TREASURE* my beer. If you make me quit it, I will CRY in my beer. Can't I pleeeease keep my beer??? I will eat less in exchange, I swear! Please? Pretty please?? PLEASE, YOU FUCKERS! PLEEEEEEEASE!!!!!!"

Poor Richard. Poor, poor Richard. He just became Homer Simpson. In print. On many bookshelves. Forever. I haven't even changed his name! I am in so much trouble! 'Cause really, what I remember him saying was something like, "Uh, guys? I have trouble falling asleep at night and a drink helps me unwind. Any chance I can be an exception to this rule?" As you can probably guess, we did not make the exception and he came around. Here's an e-mail he wrote after week 3 on the game:

*When I started this game I was suffering from a condition called sleep apnea. I've had it for years and it can be scary because you actually stop breathing while you sleep. So want to hear something crazy?? It's stopped. I have been sleeping like a baby all week. I don't know if it's the healthy eating or the weight loss or the not drinking or all of it, but I cannot express how good it feels to get a good night's sleep. And honestly, I think it has more to do with giving up the alcohol than anything else. Alcohol has been connected with sleep apnea, but I really felt like I needed to drink to fall asleep, so I never actually tried quitting before. I love you guys and I love this game. I really can't believe how great I feel.*

*—Richard*

Some of you are smiling smugly at this point. You are saying to yourselves, "Well, that may be all well and good for that Homer Simpsonesque moron named Richard. The man is a BEER drinker, for God's sake. *Of course* he should give it up. But I'm not giving up my wine. My DOCTOR told me I can have wine every night! It's good for my heart! So there! I'm keeping it, dammit!"

Well, to you I say, guess what? Your doctor said you can have wine because you wanted wine and there are studies that say wine has cardio-vascular benefits. But if you had said to your doctor, "Is there any way I can get those same benefits without the added calories and possible health detriments of alcohol?" Your doctor would have answered, "Yes!"

# The Well-documented Detrimental Effects of Alcohol on Health and Weight Loss:

- Inhibits weight loss
- Increases appetite
- Decreases inhibitions/willpower
- Adds empty calories
- Increases cortisol (a muscle-destroying hormone)
- Decreases testosterone (a muscle-building hormone)
- Decreases vitamin and mineral absorption
- Causes dehydration
- Decreases quality of sleep
- Decreases energy
- Prompts indigestion/acid reflux
- Increases risk of depression, anxiety, and insomnia
- Increases risk of liver disease, heart problems, strokes
- Increases risk of many cancers including liver, pancreatic, and breast
- Increases risk of waking up naked with an unattractive stranger

Because your goal is very likely weight loss, let's just talk for a second about how alcohol interferes with that. As I understand it, it's that your body burns the by-products of the alcohol *first* and stores whatever else you've eaten for later. Stores it for later *on your ass*. But just in case you're still more inclined to listen to an actual doctor than a TV writer who writes dialogue for fake doctors, let's hear from one! (A real doctor, not a fake one.)

• • • • • • • • • • • • • • • • • • • • • • • • • • • • • • • • • • • • • • • • •

## A word from Dr. Joseph Mercola

*Despite being widely promoted as healthy in small quantities (especially red wine), alcoholic drinks are not good for you, in any quantity.*

*The element that leads to confusion is that many people consume alcohol in the form of wine, and while there are clearly major benefits to consuming the antioxidants that are present in grape seeds and grape skins (particularly resveratrol), there are NOT benefits in the alcohol caused by fermenting the sugar in the grape pulp.*

For starters, alcohol is a neurotoxin—it can poison your brain. Alcohol can also leave you more vulnerable to various preventable cancers, can harm your body's delicate hormonal balance, and can lead to other major problems including liver damage.

Consuming large amounts of wine or any alcohol will also increase your insulin levels, which will not only raise your risk of chronic disease, it will make it much harder for you to lose weight.

In fact, insulin, stimulated by excess carbohydrates in the form of alcohol, sugar, and too many grains, is responsible for all those bulging stomachs and fat rolls in thighs and chins.

Even worse, high insulin levels suppress two other important hormones— glucagons and growth hormones—that are responsible for burning fat and sugar and promoting muscle development, respectively. So insulin from excess carbohydrates (i.e., alcohol, grains, and sugar) promotes fat, and then wards off your body's ability to lose that fat.

Alcohol, by the way, is broken down in your body into a chemical called acetaldehyde, which is the chemical responsible for hangover symptoms. When acetaldehyde reacts with the neurotransmitter dopamine, it can cause mental and emotional disturbances such as anxiety, depression, and poor concentration. If you look up the toxicology of acetaldehyde, you find that it adversely affects many tissues and organs in your body, which may play a large part in increasing the risk of so many chronic diseases and cancers.

So if you're interested in losing weight and staying healthy, eliminating alcohol, or at least limiting it significantly, is essential. And don't worry about the antioxidants you're missing; you can get plenty of those by eating fresh vegetables.

—Dr. Joseph Mercola

Dr. Mercola is the founder of Dr. Mercola's Natural Health Center, near Chicago. His Web site, Mercola.com, is the most popular natural health Web site in the world.

• • • • • • • • • • • • • • • • • • • • • • • • • • • • • • •

The last thing I'd like to say on this topic is that if your response to this rule is anything like the fictional response that I attributed to my friend Richard? If you're all, *No alcohol? NOOO alcohol??? FORGET IT. NO WAY. WHY? I'm not playing. Fuck that. No alcohol? Stupid book. Stupid game. Stupid. Forget it. I like being a fatty. I never even wanted to play anyway. No alcohol. What are you people, terrorists?* Then I'm gonna go out on a limb and suggest that you might have a bigger problem than love handles. And so I feel obliged to let you know that there is only one treatment recognized by the medical and psychiatric professions as effective in treating a physical or emotional dependence on alcohol and that treatment comes from an organization called Alcoholics Anonymous. Rumor has it it's a fun organization involving meetings spent laughing uproariously about that time you woke up in another state and had no idea how you got there.

You can find AA at www.aa.org or in your local phonebook.

*Alcoholics Anonymous is a Fellowship of Men and Women who share their experience, strength and hope with one another that they may solve their common problem and help others to recover from alcoholism. The only requirement for membership is a desire to stop drinking. There are no dues or fees for AA membership, we are self-supporting through our own contributions.*
        *—from the Preamble to the "Big Book" of Alcoholics Anonymous*

But what if you're not a drunk? What if you're just young and your social scene is built around partying? There's no twelve-step group called Party Girls and Boys Anonymous. Believe me, we get it. Az is Australian, for God's sake. His people like their beer! But if you are not as healthy as you want to be, it's imperative that you look at the fact that your whole social life is built around partying. We're not asking you to quit drinking forever— we're asking for the next four weeks. And who knows? Maybe in that time, you'll actually discover some ways to have fun and enjoy your friends that don't involve dancing on the bar or falling off it. (Man, did I love dancing on the bar and falling off it . . . Always some cute boy there to catch you. Or a filthy puddle of beer. Either way . . .) A couple of suggestions:

## Alternatives to Social Drinking

Get a group together for dance lessons. They're really fun, they burn calories, and they're not expensive (certainly no more than you'd spend on a night out at a bar).

Do as my friend Mandy recently did and organize a group to take a trapeze lesson. It's a massive adrenaline rush and a great workout to boot!

Go to an amusement park and ride roller coasters. It's my very favorite kind of adrenaline binge.

Go camping at a local beach or campground, build a fire, tell ghost stories, feel six again.

Organize a softball/soccer/touch football game in a local park. Bring a cooler of water instead of beer. Call anyone who gives you crap about the cooler a drunken loser (just for fun).

Play Truth or Dare. I don't care if you're eighty—it's a fun game.

Throw a games night and play party games like Celebrity. You'll laugh your ass off, literally. Laughing burns up to 2.5 calories per minute!

Go bowling. Suck at it. Laugh yourself silly.

Take up Los Angeles's favorite pastime: Go see a movie and then discuss all the ways you would've made it better.

Go to a baseball game. Sit in the cheap seats. Annoy fans of the opposing team. And then RUN LIKE HELL BEFORE THEY KICK YOUR ASS!

# Coffee

**The Rules:** You can have your coffee. Stop crying. We are not going to take it away. You just can't have your frothy coffee drinks.

The research on coffee and caffeine in general is really mixed. There are studies that swear it helps with weight loss and those that insist it hinders weight loss. Some say it acts as an appetite suppressant, others counter that it prompts carbohydrate cravings. We know it's a diuretic, which means it makes you pee more, but peeing out all your water isn't exactly a healthy method of weight loss. We also know it's a stimulant, which means it can increase your heart rate and blood pressure, interrupt your sleep, and cause nervousness, irritability, and anxiety.

Also euphoria.

Did I mention the euphoria?

Okay, the euphoria thing is not actually coming from scientific studies. It's coming from a study I do in my kitchen every morning. I LOVE coffee. And while science may still be debating whether or not it's good or bad for the general public, I know it's bad for me because I am actually *allergic* to it. Like, when you go to the allergist? And they poke you with the pins? I turn up allergies to dust mites and coffee. And still, I drink it every day, because that's how good the euphoria feels. Also, because it's highly physically addictive.

Still, we are not going to take it away from you (and not just because it's my personal drug of choice). We are not taking it away because it's so addictive that the sudden withdrawal from caffeine can actually defeat your ability to function in your life or enjoy any other aspect of this game.

●●●●●●●●●●●●●●●●●●●●●●●●●●●●●●●●●●●●●●●●●●●●●●●●

## Caffeine Withdrawal

●●●●●●●●●●●●●●●●●●●●●●●●●●●●●●●●●●●●●●●●●●●●●●●●

### The following are the well-documented signs and symptoms of caffeine withdrawal:

- Headache
- Fatigue
- Sleepiness/drowsiness
- Difficulty concentrating
- Irritability/decreased well-being
- Depression/Anxiety
- Flu-like symptoms including body aches and pains and nausea

- Impaired reaction time
- Meanness, crankiness, unpleasantness, bitchiness, snarkiness, weepiness, and generalized cruelty to spouses, coworkers, and pets

Fine. I made that last one up, but I bet it's true for more people than just me. 'Cause caffeine is a drug. It's a highly addictive stimulant that most of our country—adults and, sadly, kids—is strung out on. We should all take a look at our caffeine addiction and wherever we can, we should cut it back. I will tell you proudly that I am down to one cup a day and that after doing the research to write this chapter, I am more determined than ever to break my addiction.

• • • • • • • • • • • • • • • • • • • • • • • • • • • • • • • • • • • •

I'm going to reiterate that we are not going to take your coffee away from you! We are, however, going to ask you to look at how the coffee drinks you're choosing are prepared.

Why? Because a venti Caramel Frappuccino has 500 calories in it. To put that in perspective? In order to maintain a healthy weight loss, I'm supposed to be consuming about 1,500 calories a day. So one Frappuccino would be *a third of my food for the entire day.*

Believe me, we're not out to ruin your life. We really just want you to have all the information. And the sad truth is that what a lot of us order and think is coffee is really just a coffee-flavored milkshake. It's a treat. A dessert. A delicious indulgence. But it should not be a part of our daily routine.

And the thing is, it's not just the frozen frothy drinks of deliciousness that pack a caloric punch. A venti soy latte is 220 calories. Even though you are not officially counting calories on this game, you gotta know that that's a lot of liquid calories to add to your day when you're trying to lose weight. And a lot of us don't drink just one!

Remember that all weight loss boils down to energy in vs. energy burned. Energy = calories. So 220 extra calories every morning is a lot of extra energy to have to burn when you're trying to lose weight.

So drink your coffee black or lighten it with a couple of tablespoons of milk, but no more than that or you will seriously defeat your diet. (Worse, you will incur a snacking penalty and bring down your team!) And here's the thing? I used to drink and love my lattes. But when I came to understand the sad caloric realities, I switched to espresso or Café Americano (which is watered down espresso). At first, I didn't like the taste, but it took my taste buds only three days to adjust. Now, I can only enjoy my coffee black. And I don't mean that intellectually; I mean, I actually *prefer the flavor.* I guess you could say I've become a coffee purist. A coffee snob? A coffee aficionado?

How 'bout just junkie?

I think junkie pretty much sums it up.

## • • • A Tip from Az • • •

If you can't live without your morning latte or cappuccino, stick to the smallest size you can get, stick to nonfat milk, and have the drink with your first meal. You can count the nonfat milk as your carb, and then just eat some protein and healthy fat to balance it. If you want to add a little sweet, you may add a teaspoon (but no more!) of honey, maple syrup, or agave nectar (we strongly discourage artificial sweeteners because they are BAD FOR YOU).

## Diet Soda

**The Rules:** Soda and diet soda are not F.Y.T foods. Each soda or diet soda you consume carries a 10 point snacking penalty.

Soda and diet soda may be consumed without penalty on your day off and meal off. But we urge you to reconsider . . .

Before I got my very cool job writing fake medicine, I was a waitress for a good, long time. I was a waitress in Boston, I was a waitress in New York, I was a waitress in Portland, Oregon. (Sometimes, I was even a singing waitress on harbor cruise ships, but that's a whole other story.) I was a good waitress because I'm a good multitasker and I like people. Most people. I don't like people who are cheap and don't tip for good service. (And by the way? Cheap is 15 percent. For good service, please tip 20 percent. That's my little public service announcement on behalf of servers everywhere.) But my story isn't about tipping, it's about Diet Coke.

I loved Diet Coke. I was an actress back then and I used to sip my free Diet Coke at whatever restaurant I was working in and talk about how I loved it so much I would do a Diet Coke commercial *for free.* Of course, that was easy for me to say, because no one was paying me to do commercials, because mostly, I was a waitress.

The most acting I was doing in my New York days was to memorize the specials and recite them at your table, and then memorize your order without writing it down, which I considered good practice for my imaginary acting career. I was all young and carefree and I had all this room in my brain and I could just memorize the orders for a table of eight and head to the computer and get it all in, bam, bam, bam. Until one day when I couldn't. My short-term memory just *stopped working properly.* I don't know how to describe it except to say that I was twenty-two and I started having "senior moments." I would take an order, head to the computer, and by the time I got there *I would have no idea what the order was.* It was very disturbing.

I am grateful to this day that my bartender friend Corey had recently read an article about the unadvertised dangers of the artificial sweetener aspartame (NutraSweet) that I was guzzling in my Diet Coke every night.

Dude. Seriously. Go to your computer and Google the words "aspartame dangers." There is just a stunning amount of evidence as to the dangers of that chemical and the damage it does to your brain. People have died from seizures prompted by aspartame. In scientific studies, aspartame causes *holes in the brains of rats!* Aspartame causes headaches, nausea, hypertension, mood swings, depression, insomnia, memory loss . . .

Memory loss! Corey told me about the article. I quit the Diet Coke. And believe me, I was so, so, sooooo sad to quit the Diet Coke. I wanted so badly for it to not be causing my memory loss. But guess what? When I quit Diet Coke, my memory came back. Then, for good measure, and like a good junkie, I started drinking Diet Coke again, and my memory promptly went away again. So I quit for good. And I grieved. But I never went back.

I don't know why the FDA hasn't pulled the license on aspartame. I could rant some conspiracy theories at you, but I think I'm gonna let you go online and just read about it yourself because I could honestly fill a whole book on this subject alone. What I'm going to focus on here instead is one simple thing: *artificial sweeteners can cause you to gain weight*. There's a whole slew of new studies that say so. And Dr. Katz, the director of the Yale Prevention Research Center, says so in this book.

So here's the thing: Az and I were veeeeery tempted to outlaw artificial sweeteners altogether because this game is about optimizing your health, and putting chemicals into your body in place of food does not optimize your health! If you remain unconvinced, please simply look at this list:

1. Acetone
2. Acetic acid
3. Acetyl alcohol
4. Acetic anhydride
5. Ammonium chloride
6. Benzene
7. Chlorinated sulfates
8. Ethyl alcohol
9. Isobutyl ketones
10. Formaldehyde
11. Hydrogen chloride
12. Lithium chloride
13. Methanol

14. Sodium methoxide
15. Sulfuryl chloride
16. Trityl chloride
17. Toluene
18. Thionyl chloride

This is the list of chemicals used in the creation of Splenda. Y'know, the one they keep telling us is "made from sugar." Seriously. Seeeeeeeriously!!! Whatever the FDA says, whatever your doctor says, I'm asking you to answer this one question: Can you look at this list, and in your heart of hearts believe that you should be eating or drinking *anything* made from this chemical crap? Or feeding it to your *children*?

I hope you quit artificial sweeteners like a bad habit, 'cause that's what they are. But even if you're not ready to do that, we are asking you to give up sodas and diet sodas for the duration of the game, except on your meal and day off (and even then, we say, Just Say No!).

Why soda? Why not? It fills you up without satisfying your need for food. It leaves you malnourished and craving carbohydrates and sweets. And soda, whether diet or not, has recently been linked to an increase in esophageal cancer, which happens to be the disease my dad died from at fifty-six, so I take that statistic personally.

And I am now done ranting. Phew. That was exhausting, even for me.

# Frequently Asked Questions

## Alcohol

Q: What if I'm sick and I have to drink cold medicine with alcohol in it? Do I still lose points?

A: No, because we are not evil bastards. And because if you are drinking cough syrup for fun, you have bigger problems than we can address in this book.

Q: Can I take off fewer points if I drink a lower calorie alcohol?

A: Ummmmmm . . . No.

Q: What if I have two portions of alcohol on my meal off—do I still lose 25 points?

A: YES.

Q: Can I still cook with wine or sherry?

A: Yes, because the cooking burns off the metabolism-screwing part of the alcohol. But you will want to use these ingredients very lightly as they are highly caloric.

## Coffee

Q: Can I use soy creamer in my coffee?

A: Veeeery sparingly. Each tablespoon has 15 calories and a gram of fat.

Q: Can I use non-dairy creamer?

A: No. It's all sweeteners and sugar and oily non-food grossness.

Q: Our team wants to create bonus points for giving up caffeine. Can we do that?

A: It's tricky because the game depends on everyone having the same number of point-earning opportunities. If you are all drinking about the same amount of caffeine and you are all interested in kicking it, then yes, go ahead. But if not, then those of you who want to kick it can make it part of your Habit Points. As your un-healthy habit, give up caffeine. But if you are a heavy user, I suggest you wean instead of going cold turkey. Like, if you're drinking five cups a day, go to three in week 1, two in week 2, one in week 3, and none in week 4. And go you!! You rock!

## Diet Soda

Q:    Why do you go on an attack rant about my beloved artificial sweet-
      eners but not about sugar, which is also really bad for you?

A:    It is actually refined sugar that is really bad for you, as sugar found
      in fruits and vegetables and other natural foods is really healthy
      and an essential part of our daily nutritional intake. But cultur-
      ally, we tend to think of refined sugar as an unhealthy indulgence
      (which it is) while we think of artificial sweeteners as "the healthy
      alternative"—which they SO aren't. Also, refined sugar, as bad
      as it is in a thousand different ways, is at least found in nature.
      Artificial sweeteners are chemicals made in a lab. No more than
      you would go out and drink the chlorinated water from your pool
      should you be putting artificial sweeteners in your body. But you're
      right—if you want to be the healthiest you can be, you should
      eliminate all refined sugars from your life completely. All they do is
      add calories without any nutritional value at all. By the way, sugar
      is F.L.A.B.B., and you lose points for eating it.

Q:    Diet soda is my thing. I don't know how to explain it. It's my CAF-
      FEINE. It's my friend. It's my THING.

A:    I know. I've been there. And I know it's not just about the caf-
      feine. It's personal. Giving up your soda is going to be really hard
      because it's become your "I'm on a diet" status symbol. You drink
      it in public or on dates or at parties or with skinny people so you
      don't feel fat. Or so when people see your thighs they'll assume
      you're healthy or you're on a diet, and then they'll be all, "I don't
      know why she's overweight, she always drinks diet soda, must be
      her thyroid or something." We all hide behind something. Here's
      an idea: Order an iced tea with lemon (which has plenty of caf-
      feine) or a club soda with a lime. It has all the same effects—and
      no poison. Or order a green tea. Then people will KNOW you are
      a health nut, plus you get your caffeine and you may just be ward-
      ing off cancer to boot!

Q:   I can't believe what you're telling me about diet soda. I have been drinking it for years.

A:   I know. You used to go out for dinner and you'd think, *I can have those French fries as long as I get DIET soda. At least that's healthy.* (That's what I did.) And here I am telling you it's liquid poison. Well, you can be mad at me for a moment, but please don't feel stupid because you didn't know. And giant soda corporations don't want you to know. But now you know. So now you have a choice. Research it more. Or don't. Up to you.

Q:   What about natural sodas that are sweetened with juice or cane sugar—can I have those?

A:   No, because they add too many empty calories to your day, which really defeats your weight-loss goals.

Q:   So all this talk about artificial sweeteners, does that mean that on my meal off when I have dessert, I should have something with a natural sweetener in it?

A:   Yes, please!

Q:   Giving up soda sucks. I'm used to drinking three or four sodas a day. Now what am I supposed to drink?

A:   That's a lot of caffeine you're cutting out. So maybe have a little coffee or some green tea or black tea, iced or hot, to ward off caffeine withdrawal. You can stir in a small spoonful of honey or maple syrup. If you're not wanting to replace the caffeine, then just stick to water and see the water chapter for suggestions on how to spruce it up. Believe me, if you're drinking your 3 liters of water a day, you won't have much thirst left for soda.

Q:   When I stopped drinking sodas I started to get headaches. Should I be worried?

A:   That's the caffeine withdrawal. If you don't want to or can't ride it out, have a cup of black or green tea, cold or iced.

. . . . . . . . . . . . . . . . . . . . . . . . . . . . . . . . . . . . . . . . . . . . . . . .

# Play by the Rules

. . . . . . . . . . . . . . . . . . . . . . . . . . . . . . . . . . . . . . . . . . . . . . . .

### Alcohol

- You may consume one portion of alcohol during the meal off and drink freely on your day off.
- One portion equal 12 ounces of beer, 6 ounces of wine, or 1.5 ounces of hard liquor.
- If you don't make your weight-loss or fitness goal on any given week, you lose your alcohol privileges for the rest of the game.
- If you are concerned about your inability to give up alcohol but have a desire to do so, you can find support and help at www.alcoholics-anonymous.org.

### Caffeine

- Caffeine is highly addictive. Consuming less is a very good idea.
- You may add up to two tablespoons of milk to your coffee and one teaspoon of a natural sweetener without incurring a snacking penalty. But do be aware that even this much adds calories to your day—so drink your coffee or tea black if you can.
- Coffee drinks carry a hefty caloric punch. They are F.L.A.B.B. foods and should be avoided.
- If you must have a small latte in the morning, drink it with your first meal and allow the low-fat milk to be your carbohydrate for that meal.

### Diet Soda/Artificial sweeteners

- No soda or diet soda is allowed during the game except on days off and meals off.
- If you have a history of drinking a lot of soda, you may suffer caffeine withdrawal when you give it up. You might want to have a little green or black tea to ease yourself through the withdrawal.

# Chapter 15

# THE DAY OFF, THE MEAL OFF, AND 100 CALORIES OF WHATEVER YOU WANT

## (Or, Holy Nectar of the Gods, This French Toast Is *Good!*)

Disobedience . . . is man's original virtue.
It is through disobedience that progress
has been made, through disobedience
and through rebellion.

—*Oscar Wilde*

> **Rule #1:** You get one day off of every aspect of the game. Note that your food day off does not have to be the same day as your exercise day off, which can be different from your sleep day off. You can spread them out throughout the week if you choose.
>
> **Rule #2:** In addition to your food day off, you get one meal off a week. At this meal, which can last no more than 1.5 hours, you can eat whatever you want and drink one portion of alcohol without penalty.
>
> **Rule #3:** Every day, you can eat or drink 100 calories of whatever you want—*except* alcohol, soda, or diet soda—without penalty.

**I was raised** by rebels. My mother and my father were both the crunchy, hippie black sheep of their conservative families. My parents met in 1969 in Venice Beach, California. After being introduced to her over brunch at a friend's, my father showed up at my mother's door later that night and told her he'd had a dream about her when he was sixteen. Then he offered her a hit of acid.

These are my humble beginnings.

Like I said, rebels. My mother? She's the driver who pulls into the breakdown lane to speed past the rush-hour freeway traffic. She does this unapologetically and with a hint of glee in her eyes. And she once gave me a "fuzz buster" radar detector for a birthday present.

It is not in my blood to follow rules. Not societal rules. Not dietary rules. Not rules of any sort. This has served me pretty well in life, I think. Rule-followers are lovely people but they tend to wait patiently while we rebels take over the world. Hee.

My point here is, I think a HUGE part of why this game worked for me is that it allowed me—encouraged me even—to break the rules sometimes. It gave me lovely little windows of opportunity to change the daily routine. Ugh. Routine might be my least favorite word in the English language. (My friend Joan, who writes *Grey's Anatomy* with me, cannot abide the following words: "beverage," "visage," "moist," "ointment," "panties." She gets visibly upset if anyone uses them. Hilarious. But I digress . . .)

*My favorite part of the game? The day off. The day off made the whole thing possible for me. The day off is why I lost fifteen pounds and why I'm gonna keep playing and lose more.*

—Chardo, 40

I do not do well with dogma. I do not do well with laws. I do not do well with anyone who says, "You can't ever indulge if you want to lose weight!" I fundamentally rebel against that idea. And God bless Az, he came along and told me I was RIGHT!

Apparently, when you stick to the same old, same old for too long, your body gets lazy, your metabolism slows down, and it becomes harder to burn calories and lose weight. By breaking the rules once in awhile, you are saying to your metabolism, "Hey! Hey, you! Don't get too comfortable! You never know when I'm gonna hit the gas! Or the breaks! Or the gas! Or the breaks!" And now I have equated amping your metabolism with driving behind an old lady on the freeway. Which makes me happy for no good reason. I'm a little punchy. I've had too much caffeine. Whatever. The point I am trying to make here is, THIS GAME LETS YOU HAVE CANDY!!

I loooove candy.

LOVE IT.

Yum, candy.

My first ever day off of the game was in late October, and I ate Halloween candy for breakfast.

Nine pieces.

I also ate it for snacks, for lunch, and for dinner, in addition to French toast, French fries, ice cream, and pizza. You think I'm kidding. You have noticed, perhaps, that I have a tendency to exaggerate; a flair for the dramatic. Yes, I do, but in this case, I'm stating the facts. I wish I could stand before you a beacon of health and moderation. I wish I could say simply and melodically, "It was so delightful on that first day off to enjoy a small bit of chocolate after my slightly larger than usual salad." But if I were that person, I would not have been fifty pounds overweight to begin with. Plus, I would have large, bright, white wings and I would happily fly to work each day and spare Mother Earth the emissions from my zippy hybrid vehicle.

What I *can* say, in all honesty, is that I do not recommend that you do as I did on that first day off. As it turns out, this kind of eating has a detrimental effect on weight loss. Also on sanity. What's funny is, I wasn't even feeling all that deprived by my day off. I didn't even crave most of those foods. But the theory I embraced was, *Can't have it for the rest of the week! Must shove it all in now!*

The one really nice benefit to that sugar and fat binge was that I was so sick by the end of the day, I didn't want a single gross thing for the rest of the week. By next day, I was eager and happy to be back on a healthy eating plan. I was also cranky, moody, headachey, tired, and hungover. No booze necessary.

Like I said, I don't recommend it. As it turns out, moderation, even on the day off, is key. Which is not to say you shouldn't have Halloween candy for breakfast. Halloween candy for breakfast is delightful. But maybe the crazy stops there.

## Step Up Your Game!

If you are worried about undoing your good work with your day or meal off, consider these tactics:

Take a different exercise day off from your food day off! By exercising on your food day off, you keep your metabolism kicking through the extra calories. You also remind yourself of your commitment to your health.

Drink all your water on your food day off! The water will sate your appetite so you don't overeat and will help your metabolism do its job.

Eat F.L.A.B.B foods for only one meal on your food day off. For the rest of the day, stick to foods on the F.Y.T. list and just don't worry about timing/portions. You'll definitely feel healthier on the morning after if you play this way!

Forgo the alcohol. I've never seen Az take a drink of alcohol. Which is not to say he doesn't like it—he's Australian! But his body is his priority and alcohol functions like poison in the body. If weight loss is your goal, it's the first thing to skip!

At your meal off, have bread, wine, OR dessert. Don't have all three.

## The 100 Calories of Whatever You Want Rule

We added the 100 calories of whatever rule to help balance the "gotta get it all in now" panic. And you know what? It really works. Knowing I can have a bite or two of anything I want every day lets me relax on my day off and not eat like a prisoner who was just set free. Az wants me to point out that it also teaches those of us who have trouble with moderation (that would be me, not him) to *practice moderation*. Apparently, it is a muscle that can be developed like any other. And I will admit that knowing I get only a hundred calories of a thing does prompt me to slow down and reeeeealllly enjoy it.

This rule is also in place so that you never have to be the person at a birthday party who can't taste the cake. Or the person in cooking class who can't taste the ice cream you just made from scratch. Or the person on Halloween who can't have a piece of candy. Game on or game off, life is for living.

## Step Up Your Game!

Consider starting your game on a Wednesday! By playing Wednesday to Wednesday, you will feel far less license to over-indulge on your day off. Why? Because when you start on a Monday, you will weigh in on the Saturday or Sunday morning *before* your day off. When you start on a Wednesday, you will take a weekend day off and then you will have to weigh in only three days later, on Wednesday morning. You won't have a whole week to recover from your day off indulging! Weigh in fear might give you the added push you need to embrace moderation on your day off!

There are, believe it or not, days when I forget about this rule entirely. But there are also days when I can't live without a York Peppermint Patty after lunch, and even if I can, I don't want to. There are only 40 calories in the little ones. So I get to eat TWO. And when you know you get only two, you chew them slowly, taste them fully, and actually feel satisfied afterward. (Whereas, in the past, I might have popped eight of them in while working and chatting and not even tasted most of them. And then maybe felt a little sick after.)

This rule entitles us to culinary delights. But because 100 calories of culinary delights come in pretty small packages, it also encourages us to get present with our food, which many experts say is the ultimate key to losing weight and keeping it off. (And, by the way, because you can't generally measure calories in a birthday cake or homemade ice cream, a good rule on this is the *rule of thumb*—no larger a portion than the size of your thumb and you should be within your 100-calorie limit.)

Please note that the only things you may NOT consume under this rule are soda, diet soda, and alcohol. Why? Because alcohol wreaks havoc with your metabolism's ability to do its job. And soda and diet soda are largely responsible for the obesity epidemic in this country. Our hope is to break you of the soda habit completely! (Or at the very least make you save them for your day and/or meal off.)

> *I looooove the 100 calories rule! Love it love it love it love it love it. No other diet I've tried lets me eat my Smarties and not feel guilty!! So on other diets, I obsess about them. Now I don't obsess, I just enjoy the heck out of them—and I keep losing weight!*
>
> —J.K., 35

## The Meal Off

Speaking of the meal off, it has the same antideprivation effect as the 100 calories. The meal off also allows you to go out with friends once a week and not have to be "the dieter." Or it allows you to indulge in a coworker's birthday cake at the office. Or it allows you to cook pancakes on a Thursday morning for no good reason.

But aside from the psychological effects, the meal off and day off actually serve a physiological purpose, which is to boost your caloric intake so that your body doesn't adjust to the calorie deficit and hit a plateau. What does that mean?

It means that even if you are, unlike me, a person who thrives on routine, you should still boost your calories twice a week. Do you have to eat candy and crap? No. And I will admit that you will be much healthier for not eating it. But you must still bring your calories up to non-dieting levels twice a week to avoid the dreaded "plateau" effect that many people experience when dieting. (For more on this, see Chapter 16, Troubleshooting.)

### • • • A Tip from Az • • •

A lot of folks wonder if they really need to take the Day Off. My answer is, absolutely they do. It is not a day of bingeing! It is not a day of insanity (as Krista learned the hard way). It is a day of rest—a day when you don't have to think about the rules, don't have to think about the "diet," don't have to think.

The body, mind, and spirit really do require a day of rest in order to function at maximum intensity for the rest of the week. So enjoy the day! And yeah, even indulge a little (because the calorie boost really helps your metabolism thrive!). Learn to enjoy the great pleasures of life—some of which come in the form of food. Skip the cheap candy bar (unless a cheap candy bar is truly your favorite food) and try a really good panna cotta or crème brûlée (my favorite poison).

And then practice the art of forgoing regret!

Guilt-free indulgence is one of the truly happiest side effects of playing this game!

The other really nice thing about the Day Off, the Meal Off, and the 100 Calories of Whatever is that they teach those of us who have been taught to think in extremes that it doesn't have to be all or nothing. How many times have you started your day with good intentions (diet-wise) and then eaten a donut at the office and thought, "Well fuck it. This day is a waste. May as well go to McDonald's for lunch and eat a pint of ice cream for dinner." Turns out, that's not true. Turns out, calories are cumulative, and just because you ate a donut, the day is not a total waste. People who are naturally sane around food already understand this. I did not. So these "rules," these little indulgences, teach us—train us, even—that it's possible to eat the donut and get right back on the healthy train for the rest of the day. (*Even if the donut is a snacking penalty, you can get back on the game for the rest of the day!*)

What I love about this rule, and about this game, is that it acknowledges what no other "diet" I've tried acknowledges—that sometimes we need to indulge. That all of us, even the sanest eaters I know, use food emotionally. We use it to quell sadness, we use it to celebrate success, we use it for many reasons other than sustenance, and that isn't such a terrible thing. It's only a terrible thing—for our bodies, for our minds, for our spirits—when we use food that way all the time. When we regularly use food to *not feel* our feelings, to stuff them down, that's a serious problem (and a sign that maybe we need more help than any diet book can provide). For more on this, let's turn to a professional.

• • • • • • • • • • • • • • • • • • • • • • • • • • • • • • • • • • • • •

# A word on emotional eating from therapist Jennifer Burton

*Eating for comfort is not always a problem. The problem arises when we are engaging in emotional eating on a regular basis, and doing so without awareness. Often we eat instead of letting ourselves feel whatever created the urge to eat in the first place. Some common emotions we tend to use food to avoid are anger, sadness, grief, embarrassment, loneliness, and frustration (and these are just a few). These feelings can arise from current life stress, or they can be a result of past issues bubbling to the surface.*

*I would encourage inserting a pause (at least 5 minutes) prior to eating the snack you're reaching for. During this pause, sit down, take a couple of breaths, and check in with your body. What do you notice inside? Remember that we wouldn't know what our feelings are if our body wasn't giving us clues (for example, throat tightening and tears can signify sadness, flushing and tension can signify anger, and so on), and for everyone the signs of emotions can be different. By checking in, you will get a sense of what your own body's clues are. Once you notice what you are feeling and sensing inside, you might journal about what's coming up and allow yourself to feel more deeply into it. This process of pausing, checking in, writing, and feeling will at least give you more awareness, and if you still choose the comfort food, you'll be doing so mindfully.*

*In addition, there are many other forms of comfort other than food (honestly). The feelings coming up for you may arise out of an unmet need. "I need a friend"; "I need rest"; "I need a hug." Make a list of healthy resources that provide comfort. This list can include friends, pets, books and poems, hobbies, dancing or exercise, taking a bath, or even a stuffed animal you might still have around. By having a written list handy, you can decide to use healthy resources instead of eating. One caveat: when unmet needs come from unresolved past issues, you may need to seek professional help to address and heal those wounds. A trusted therapist can be helpful as you move down your path to a more balanced and fulfilling life (not to mention an added resource!)*

*Jennifer Burton, MFT, CEAT, therapist specializing in trauma and other life issues*
*www.jenniferburtonmft.com*

• • • • • • • • • • • • • • • • • • • • • • • • • • • • • •

As a side note, I feel I must add that if you are a person with an eating addiction then this rule might not work for you. Just as an alcoholic can't have *any* alcohol or risk triggering a physical allergy and a mental obsession, a food addict has to live by different rules. If you think you're a food addict, please seek help. They have twelve-step groups that are free (like Overeaters Anonymous) or you can get therapy or help from an eating-disorders specialist. (See the section on eating disorders at the end of Chapter 16.)

# Frequently Asked Questions

Q: I'm going on vacation. Can I skip my day off this week so I can have an extra day when I'm away?

A: No, I'm sorry, you can't. You'll be screwing yourself this week by not giving your metabolism the calorie boost it needs and you'll be screwing yourself next week by having two days off. But you can savor your meal off and your day off and enjoy the hell out of your vacation anyway!

Q: I ate WAY too much on my day off and then had to have Tums the next day. Is there a penalty for that?

A: Yes, the penalty is the physical pain you put yourself in! The reward is that hopefully you've learned from this experience. And by the way, Tums have 5 calories apiece and are not all-natural, so go easy. (Papaya is a good natural remedy for heartburn.)

Q: I LOVE the day off. I mean really, really love it. So much so that I have a hard time getting motivated the next day to get back in the game. Any advice?

A: Read the last chapter of this book. It's a little pep talk just for you.

Q: Whyyyyyyy can't I have my diet soda every day?? It has NO CALORIES!!

A:   Please reread Chapter 14 about what you're doing to your body when you drink that shit. (For starters, the sodium in the soda bloats you and the chemical sweeteners make you crave sweets and carbs. And that's just for starters.) I really hope you will just quit it cold turkey. But if you can't or don't want to, you can still mainline the crack on your day off and meal off.

Q:   I admit that I'm a control freak. I like limitations—they make me feel safe, so the day off kind of messes with my head. Can I skip it?

A:   Boy, do I not relate. But okay, yeah, stick to F.Y.T. foods on your day off and just eat a little more of them. It actually doesn't take that much extra to give your metabolism a boost.

Q:   I LOVE the day off rule, but I can't stop my mind from telling me that I'm doing something wrong when I bump up my calories. I know it's okay, but I still feel guilty. Any advice of what to do in those moments?

A:   Guilt is a waste of energy. If you persist in feeling guilty, do as the control freak does and stick to F.Y.T. foods on your day off—just eat more of them.

Q:   Do you lose points if you don't take a day off?

A:   No, but you are actually setting yourself back. Do as the biblical God did and take a freakin' day off! You've earned it!

• • • • • • • • • • • • • • • • • • • • • • • • • • • • • • • • • • • • • • •
## Play by the Rules
• • • • • • • • • • • • • • • • • • • • • • • • • • • • • • • • • • • • • • •

- You get one day off a week from all aspects of the game.
- Your food day off can be different from your water day off, which can be different from your exercise day off, etc.
- On your food day off you may consume alcohol but please don't binge.

- You get one two-hour long meal off a week as well.
- At your meal off, you may also consume one portion of alcohol.
- You may consume 100 calories of whatever you want—except alcohol, soda, or diet soda—each day.

Chapter 16

# TROUBLESHOOTING

## (Or, WTF Am I Doing Wrong?!)

No problem is so big or so complicated that it
can't be run away from.

—*Charles Schulz*

I gained two pounds last week, while playing the game. First time ever that I've gained weight while playing. Am I pissed? No. Am I surprised? No. Am I irritated? Mmm . . . Not really. I knew it was a bad week. I knew it was a bad week because I had a headache that was so bad, I couldn't exercise *at all*. I had a headache that was so bad, in fact, that my doctor ordered a head CT. *A head CT.*

On *Grey's Anatomy*, when we have the doctors order head CTs, that doesn't usually go too well for the patient. There is almost always a tumor, or an aneurysm, or some rare condition that requires McDreamy to remove half of someone's brain. Picture me, at my doctor's office, explaining the exact combination of pounding and throbbing and pulsing in my skull that sets in at 11 a.m. every day. Now, the doctor I work with in the writer's room had said it was probably sinusitis. So I'm expecting some antibiotics and a pat on the back. And instead, it goes like this:

HIM: I've never heard of a sinus headache that throbs the way you're describing. And I've never heard of a sinus headache that you don't feel upon awakening. I'm gonna want to get a scan.

ME: I'm sorry, what? A scan? You mean like a CT?

HIM (all casual-like): Yeah.

CUT TO:

Me, driving to Beverly Hills, picturing saying a sobbing goodbye to my child and my husband, then watching my funeral as a ghost. *Hmm . . . who would be there? Who would be crying?* ME! I WOULD!! I WOULD BE A GHOST AND I WOULD BE FUCKING CRYING AT MY OWN FUNERAL!!! I'M TOO YOUNG TO DIE!!!!

CUT TO:

Me, after the head CT, talking to the technician who ran it.

ME: Are you looking at pictures of my brain?

TECH: Yup.

ME: How does it look?

TECH: Not allowed to comment.

ME (batting my lashes): Oh, I know. I know officially you're not allowed
     to comment, but you guys do this all day. You know more than the
     doctors.

TECH: Not allowed to comment, sorry.

ME: What if I told you I'm the head writer at *Grey's Anatomy*?

TECH: (laughs)

ME: No, seriously, I am. And I'm soooo curious to see what you guys
     actually do for a living.


Turns out it was sinusitis. The nice tech showed me on the scan.

So, I gained two pounds. And the almost-dying scenario that wasn't
real but felt real for about an hour? Puts that in perspective. I also know
exactly why I gained weight: because I ate the amount of food I'm supposed to eat if I'm exercising every day and I did not exercise even one
day. I should've cut my portions back, but I was busy and hungry and not
really playing as passionately as I usually do because of the headache. A
little weight gain—not so surprising. And this week, with the headache
gone, I stepped it up and lost three pounds.

That's what I love about having all the information. I never have to wonder why. If I gained weight, it's because I ate more energy than I burned.
When I'm ready to lose it, I have to burn more than I eat. The end.

So why didn't I quit when my headache was so bad that I was losing
my exercise points every day? Because even when I am playing this game
at 80 percent or 70 percent or 60 percent, I am living a whole lot healthier
life than I am when I'm not playing. And my commitment is to my health
first, then to my team. And I always choose to play with people who get
that and support that and play the same way. I would NEVER want a
teammate to drop out because an illness was prompting a point loss. I
would want them to play to the best of their ability (because the sleep and
the water and healthy eating is the fastest way to recover from illness) and
trust that someone on the other team is likely going through something
similar. (Hmmm. Does that count as schadenfreude?)

In preparation for writing this book, we did a lot of focus groups. Which means we played a lot of games, we had our friends play a lot of games, and we had a lot of strangers play a lot of games and report back to us.

Here's what we found: Most people lost a bunch of weight the first week (a couple of real pounds and then a bunch of water weight) and then lost weight again in week two. In week three, about 25 percent of players didn't lose weight. And then in week four, they lost weight again.

So what were those 25 percent doing? Mostly, they had gotten lazy with their portion control and with their food choices. (E.g.: They were eating in restaurants and paying no attention to how the meals were prepared.) Some of them were lacking integrity (claiming points they had "only sort of" earned). Some of them had gotten sick or injured and quit or "sort of" quit.

Basically, they had all slipped in their attention to detail, and when they refocused, the weight started to drop off again. I know. I know you want to think this isn't you. When our computers crash, we all want to blame the computer. But just as 90 percent of the time "computer error" is actually human error, 90 percent of the time, when your game isn't getting you the results you desire, the problem isn't with the game—it's with how you're playing it.

## Step Up Your Game!

Keep a food diary. It's simple. Just write down everything you eat. In one major study, it was found that keeping a food journal can double a dieter's weight loss! It doesn't have to be a formal journal—at each meal, you can send yourself an e-mail, a text message, or just jot it down on a Post-it Note. The point is just to write it all down, which keeps you ever more aware and fully accountable.

## Overindulging—like, waaaaay overindulging

On one particularly memorable occasion, my friend Adam proudly went out for a *sixteen-course meal off*—and then had the gall to wonder why he didn't lose weight that week! Which is generally the other thing that was happening for the non–weight-losers—they were going hog wild on their day off and meal off. And by hog wild I mean they were *undoing* their dieting for the rest of the week. The day off and meal off are in place for two reasons: One, so your body doesn't adjust to the calorie deficit and slow your metabolism accordingly. And two, so you don't feel overly deprived. But all you're supposed to be doing is bringing your calorie intake back up to non-dieting levels. You are not supposed to be bringing it up to *bingeing* levels. You are not supposed to be eating seven days worth of crap in one crazy day of non-stop eating. That's not a day off. That's a day of insanity. This game is about optimizing your health. Binge eating, even one day a week, does not optimize your health. And if that's what you're doing, you need to stop. (And if you can't stop, you should see the section on eating disorders at the end of this chapter and consider seeking help.)

> *I was so frustrated at first—all of my friends were losing weight, but I wasn't, and I had the most to lose! Then I did the actual math and figured out that I ate over 10,000 calories one Sunday. 'Cause I'm that kinda guy. Anyway, when I did the math I saw that on my day off, I was undoing every bit of good I was doing during the week. So I adopted a little more moderation on the day off and voilà. Fifteen pounds off and counting . . .*
>
> —Adam, 38

## Mountain Climbing

The other thing that players have run into, usually after playing the game two or three times, is a marked slowing down of weight loss. Usually, it happens to people with not a lot of weight left to lose. And it's what in dieting vernacular is known as hitting a plateau.

## • • • A Tip from Az • • •

Every dieter at one time or another will hit the dreaded weight-loss plateau. Your body is simply attempting to protect you by slowing your metabolism down to match the amount of energy you're consuming, so you won't waste away. This is why we include the meal off and day off—to boost your calories back up and keep your metabolism burning at its maximum capacity. Unfortunately a meal or day off may not be enough, depending on how long you've been dieting. If you've hit a plateau, I suggest boosting your calories back up for a couple of days or even a full week to reboot your metabolism. Your weight might just pop up slightly for these few days but your body will be burning at a much higher level.

Please do not see a plateau as a sign to decrease your portions/calories even more. This is not only dangerous; it's detrimental to your health and weight-loss goals! If you are playing all out, then the deficit you are on is *enough*. To cut your food intake back further is a sure way to disaster as you will be depleting your body of vital nutrients it needs. When you've hit a plateau, your body has simply adjusted to your new routine, so it is time to change things up. What changes can you make?

- Change your exercise routine. If you usually jog, try swimming, or cycling—anything that will change the way your body is working.
- Add strength training to your weekly exercise routine. Working your muscles will help boost your metabolism.
- Change up your diet. Are you eating the same things every single day? Startle your body by eating different foods and adding or decreasing your protein one day and your carbs the next.

*Az put me on a meal plan and I was losing weight and it felt great so I figured why not eat even less and lose even more? And then I lost no weight that week. When Az found out what I'd done, he yelled at me in that cute Australian way he has that makes you feel like he's mocking and loving you even when he yells. I ate more the next week and, presto, change-o, my weight loss resumed. The moral of this story? Listen to Az. And oh yeah, don't starve yourself.*

—Cristine, 32

## Blooooooooating

The fact remains, if you're playing all out, you'll almost always lose weight consistently and with relative ease. Still, if you're playing all out and reading this chapter in desperation, then you should know about the other exceptions we've found that may mess with the numbers on your scale (and not in a good way). They are:

- Morning after meal off or day off
- Constipation
- Menstruation

After a meal off or day off, you are usually carrying some extra water weight because usually, you ate something salty or oily or sugary or you drank alcohol. Your body has an adjustment period when it retains some extra water. Just stay consistent with your game and the scale should be where you want it within a day or two.

Similarly, and now I'm speaking to the ladies, when you have or are about to have your period, you tend to carry some extra water weight. Nothing to be done about that. Don't panic. Just notice the increase in weight, keep playing all out, and it will regulate.

And, finally, when you are constipated, you tend to carry some extra . . . er . . . poo weight. Eew. Gross. Can't believe I just wrote that. But I seriously know people who've lost two or three pounds after y'know . . .

in the hospital they call it "evacuating the bowels" but there's just no good way to say it. Birthing a poo baby?

That said, DO NOT ABUSE LAXATIVES TO MAKE WEIGHT! This is an integrity issue. If you take a laxative because you want to make your weigh-in, *you lose all your points for the week!!* Don't do it. It's bad for your health and bad for your game. (If you're tempted, see the section in the back of this chapter about eating disorders and get some help.) Here instead are ten suggestions about how to avoid this problem before it starts or to relieve it naturally . . .

• • • • • • • • • • • • • • • • • • • • • • • • • • • • • • • • • • • • • • • • • •
## 10 Tips to Avoid or Relieve Constipation
• • • • • • • • • • • • • • • • • • • • • • • • • • • • • • • • • • • • • • • • • •

1. Include more fruits in your daily diet.
2. Chew your food thoroughly.
3. Eat steamed, fresh vegetables.
4. Drink a glass of warm water with lemon juice and a pinch of salt upon waking.
5. Avoid eating fried food, frozen food, and food or drinks with preservatives.
6. Always go to the bathroom when you have the urge. (Don't "hold it" for later.)
7. Exercise first thing in the morning.
8. Stretch your body upon awakening. Specifically, try twisting poses (yoga) to stimulate the bowel.
9. Squat for 10 minutes upon awakening. (You can do this watching TV or playing with your baby.)
10. When sitting on the toilet, place your feet on a small step stool, which makes everything move a little easier.

## Eating what's right but feeling all wrong

Finally, being an alternative medicine girl (my acupuncturist has *never* sent me for an unnecessary head CT), I feel I must add this: People have food sensitivities. Food sensitivities are not quite allergies—but they can wreak havoc with your body's ability to function optimally (i.e., your metabolism). Sensitivities to wheat and dairy are very common but there are many others. (I personally do not feel at all well when I eat any animal flesh other than fish.) Since I'm not actually a doctor (as much as the other *Grey's* writers and I like to pretend we are), let's hear from Dr. Leo Galland, who is, quite simply, awesome.

• • • • • • • • • • • • • • • • • • • • • • • • • • • • • • • • • • • • • • • • • • • • • • • • •

## A word from Dr. Leo Galland

*Food sensitivities have an important impact on weight loss and on overall health. About half the population has them. Although food sensitivity takes many forms, most are related to the <u>protein</u> content of specific foods. Some people thrive on a high protein intake. They need meat and perhaps dairy. I call them hunter/herder types. Others thrive on a vegetarian, plant-based diet, with little or no animal protein. Still others are intolerant of a specific food protein, such as the casein in milk or the gluten in wheat. At least 2 million Americans are gluten intolerant. There are no perfect lab tests for food sensitivity. Once you've eliminated sugar and junk foods, which nobody thrives on, you can usually determine your food sensitivities by observing how you feel after different types of meals. Do you have fatigue, headaches, bloating, aches and pains? Do you feel swollen and heavy? Do these symptoms come and go? When are they worst? Early in the morning . . . think about what you ate last night. In mid-afternoon . . . what did you eat for lunch? If you eat a steak, do you feel energetic and strong or sleepy and fuzzy-headed? If you eat only salad, do you feel refreshed and light or shaky and weak? Does a hearty whole grain bread leave you feeling satisfied or bloated? Answering these questions can not only help you feel your best, it can help you achieve your optimal* *weight. Whenever I see a patient who can't lose weight on a healthy diet, I look for food sensitivities. Ninety percent of the time, identifying them allows for weight loss to proceed as expected.*

*Leo Galland, MD, author of* The Fat Resistance Diet
*www.fatresistancediet.com*

• • • • • • • • • • • • • • • • • • • • • • • • • • • • • • • • • •

It comes back to this: Pay attention to your body. Notice how you feel and then try eliminating the foods that make you feel like crap and see if that act alone doesn't increase your metabolism and speed up your weight loss.

And, of course, before embarking on this game, you should've gone to your doctor to confirm that you are in good health. There are a variety of health conditions—from heart problems to thyroid problems to kidney problems to gland problems—that can interfere with your body's ability to shed weight. If you feel like you're doing everything right and nothing is working, get a thorough checkup!

The final thing I want to say here is that if you don't lose weight one week, it's not the end of the world. This game/diet/lifestyle change is meant to be both healthy and *fun*. Even if you didn't make weight, your health has no doubt improved if you are playing this game all out. And hopefully, you're having fun while improving your health, which is huge! I'm not saying your weight loss isn't important. I'm just asking you to look for what you can change to improve that aspect of your game while still giving yourself credit for your hard work. I'm asking you to please not beat yourself up. Brain tumors and aneurysms and needing half your brain removed, that's serious and scary. While I did not enjoy the few hours I had to ponder those possibilities in my life last week, I am grateful for the perspective those hours gave me when I got on the scale at the end of the week and the numbers were up. So let's get you some perspective right now.

# GET A PEN!

Write down ten things in your life for which you are truly grateful. If you're really feeling low, start with the basics like "My functioning limbs" and work your way up to "My family loves me." The exercise will give you perspective without an unnecessary CAT scan of your brain. Come on. Really, really. Get a pen. Riiiiiiiiight . . . NOW!

_____

_____

_____

_____

_____

_____

_____

_____

_____

_____

## A Word About Eating Disorders

This country has an epidemic of eating disorders. There is a part of me that is reticent to attach my voice to a "diet" of any sort because I have so many friends—men and women—who have suffered greatly from the psychological effects of living in a society that puts such a high premium on skinniness. Not even beauty. Beauty's its own thing. Beauty is subjective. Skinniness is just skinniness. Even if you think that some of these too-skinny celebrities look pretty gross and like a bag of bones, as long as *People* magazine puts them on the cover in couture and holds them up as an ideal, we are all affected.

That said, I play this game because it helps me feel better. It helps me feel more emotionally balanced, more physically able, and more capable of taking control of my own health. If it's doing the opposite for you, stop playing and consider seeking help. If you have a history of eating disorders, or a current problem with an eating disorder, I have tremendous compassion for your struggle and I hope you seek treatment and I wish you health. Google the words "eating disorder help" and you will find many programs and resources to help you.

• • • • • • • • • • • • • • • • • • • • • • • • • • • • • • • • • • • • • • • •

## A word from eating disorder specialist Michella Fiordaliso Eating Disorder Warning Signs

*In an image-crazed society it's virtually impossible to never think about your weight or diet. However, there is a place where normal preoccupation can become an unhealthy obsession. Do you . . .*

- *Feel paranoid about eating?*
- *Sneak or hide food?*
- *Eat in secret?*
- *Have constant thoughts about food?*
- *Have body dysmorphic syndrome—a perception of your body that isn't accurate? For example, seeing yourself as fat even though the scale doesn't indicate that.*
- *Feel anxious or depressed about your relationship to food or conversely use food to manage anxiety and depression?*
- *Purge: use laxatives or vomit?*
- *Have two sets of eating habits (one for in public and one for in private)?*
- *Exercise excessively?*
- *Binge eat?*
- *Resort to extreme measures (double up on workouts, starve yourself, purge)?*
- *Talk about food and weight all the time?*
- *Weigh yourself multiple times a day?*
- *Eat the same foods every day?*
- *Take stimulants (including overconsuming caffeinated beverages)?*
- *Always find yourself on a diet even since you were a child?*
- *Feel like there are two separate people in you (one who wants to eat well and one who tells you to forget about it and eat what you want)?*

*If you find yourself experiencing any of the traits above, consider seeking therapy or a support group to understand your relationship to food and how to have greater peace of mind around eating.*

*Michelle Fiordaliso, MSW, Clinical Director, Shrink Yourself*
*www.shrinkyourself.com*

• • • • • • • • • • • • • • • • • • • • • • • • • • • • • • •

# Frequently Asked Questions

Q:  What if I have my period on weigh-in day and I KNOW I would've made weight if I didn't?

A:  Women get a once-a-game period pass. Which means you don't have to make weight the week you have your period—but you do have to make weight *for both weeks* the following week. And what I mean by that is, if you weigh 150 and your goal weight for the week is 148.5 and you have your period and don't make your goal, you get a pass. BUT the next week, you must weigh in at 147—which means you actually did lose the weight the week of your period even though the scale didn't reflect it and you also lost your weight this week. Otherwise, you don't get your bonus points for the week of your period.

Q:  Yeah, but what if I have my period the last week of the game?

A:  Ideally, you shouldn't time your game this way. But if you must, then you can ask your team and opponents for a few extra days at the end before final scores are calculated. If the game is tight, whether or not you make your bonus will make a difference, so in the interest of good sportsmanship (sportswomanship?) they should give you the extra time.

Q:  I'm a guy—is there some equivalent of a "period pass" for me?

A:  Shut up and be grateful that you don't hemorrhage from your penis once a month. Ass.

Q:    My husband is not playing the game and he keeps bringing home
      high-calorie food like pizza and fast food. I've asked him not to,
      but he just says he can do whatever he wants. I think he's jealous
      of my new body. I don't want to cause a fight, but don't know how
      to handle this.

A:    Sadly, your husband is right. He isn't supportive. He isn't maybe
      the best husband in the world when it comes to your diet. But
      he's right. He can do whatever he wants. And so can you. You
      can't control his choices—but you can control yours. And you
      can choose compassion. Maybe he's feeling threatened by your
      new body, by your new lifestyle, by your new you. Maybe he was
      comfortable and happy with the old you, even if you weren't. And
      maybe he doesn't know how to communicate any of this. So I
      would suggest that even though your impulse is to smack him
      upside the head, maybe try the opposite and tell him you love him
      a lot. Tell him frequently and lovingly and passionately. Instigate a
      tickle match. Instigate sex. Also? Leave the house when the pizza
      arrives. And if you can't leave the house, at least leave the room.
      Go and do something healthier than sitting around smelling pizza
      and resenting him. Don't spend your precious energy trying to
      change him. Just love him, and keep changing you. Eventually, he
      may just decide to join you.

Q:    I have a group of friends who are all overweight. We used to do
      lots of eating outings together, but now that I'm playing the game,
      things have changed. They don't want to play and it seems like the
      more weight I lose the less they want to do with me. I don't want
      to lose these friendships. What should I do?

A:    Friendships change and fall away for a thousand reasons. You are
      prioritizing your health! If your friends can't support that, you
      have to ask if these are really healthy friendships that you want
      to hold on to. If they are, then maybe you just need to reach out.
      Pick your favorite friend and say, "Sally! I miss you! And I'm play-
      ing this game so I can't do our old restaurant thing. Wanna just

come over for a cup of tea and catch up?" Maybe she does. And if she doesn't, you've learned something. Most of my close friends have been my close friends for nearly twenty years. But a couple of friends have fallen away in recent years and when that happens it makes me really sad. And that's when my therapist has had to remind me that there is a difference between *best* friends and *old* friends. If these are truly your best friends, they will support you in your journey to improve your health.

Q: I SWEAR I am playing all out! I SWEAR I am doing everything you say to do!! But I am not losing weight!!! Heeeeelp!!!!!

A: Okay, I can help. The help goes like this: Try counting calories, because if you are doing everything right, then something in what or how much you're eating is wrong. So go to our Web site, www .thegameondiet.com, and enter your weight and height and age. The site will then do a little math for you and tell you tell you how many calories you should be eating to lose weight if you are doing the HIIT exercise three times a week and 20 minutes of moderate exercise another three times a week. On our Web site, you will also find a source to help you count calories. Do it VIGILANTLY for a week. Pay attention to exactly what and how much you can eat to stay under this number and I will be stunned if you don't lose weight! Full disclosure: I count calories! Why? Because my food sensitivities make it hard for me to consistently eat all the lean protein we recommend. And it's the lean protein that really helps keep the calorie count down. So in the beginning, I played the way we are recommending you play. But after a while, when I got tired of all that protein, I started to count calories. Counting calories, while it sounds very eighties and Richard-Simmons-in-a-unitard, is actually the best way to have all the information. Because the rule is this: If you burn more energy than you consume, you will lose weight. And counting calories lets you know exactly how much energy you're consuming! You don't have to do it forever, just try it for a week or two—see if it doesn't change what/how much you eat and kick your weight loss into high gear!

Q: Sometimes when I don't make my weight I get so depressed, even if I know why. What should I do?

A: Reread the list of things you're grateful for. Then make a new list, adding fifty more things. *The air. The sky. My television. The fact that I live in a free country. The fact that women get to vote* . . . FIFTY THINGS THAT HAVE NOTHING TO DO WITH THE SIZE OF YOUR ASS. Also talk about your feelings to a friend. Sometimes it really helps just to say it out loud.

## Play by the Rules

- When you burn more energy than you eat, you will lose weight.
- If you don't make weight, don't beat yourself up. Take a breath, and then look at your portion sizing, food choices, and exercise. Make adjustments the following week.
- The day off and meal off are in place to keep your metabolism burning at optimum speed and to keep you from feeling deprived.
- Bingeing on your day off or meal off can sabotage your entire week and result in weight gain.
- The morning after a day off or meal off your body is adjusting and may carry some extra water weight, so don't panic. (You may want to skip weighing yourself this day.)
- You will carry extra weight if you are constipated or premenstrual. Again, don't panic. Just notice and keep playing all out.
- Food sensitivities are common and can affect your body's ability to function optimally. If you suspect you are sensitive to certain foods, try eliminating these foods from your diet and see how it affects your weight loss.
- If you've reached a plateau, try mixing it up by doing different exercises or changing the amount of calories you eat per meal (while still keeping within the rules of the game).

- If playing this game is triggering obsessive, unhealthy behaviors and awakening an eating disorder, please stop playing and seek support.
- Even if you have a "bad" week, you are still improving your health. Be sure to give yourself credit for what you have done and all the hard work and courage it takes to play this game. You rock!

Chapter 17

# POSTGAME WRAP-UP

## (Or, I Am Liking This New Ass of Mine.)

If you want a happy ending,
that depends, of course,
on where you stop your story.
—*Orson Welles*

**I'm on the** East Coast at a reunion of my husband's family, and my husband and baby and in-laws have been out playing on the beach in Cape Cod all week while I sit holed up in the dark writing because I'm up against some pretty tight deadlines. I love writing but I love my family and the beach even more and so I've been a little sad about missing out. And so I have been comforting myself with donuts. Also, I have been consuming copious amounts of coffee, not stopping to exercise or getting up to stretch, not drinking enough water . . . Pretty much every healthy habit I have ever learned while playing the game has gone to hell this week while I write the book about the game. Ironic, no?

My husband's cousin's lovely wife, Enid, walked in this morning and said, "How are you?" and I said, "I don't know. Fine, I guess. I'm fine. Panicking, but fine. My deadline is hurtling toward me like some unseen force of darkness while everyone plays on the beach but I guess, y'know, whatever, I'm fine."

Poor Enid. She smiled gently and asked if there was anything she could do for me. And I realized that unless she could go buy me a little slice of sanity at a corner market, no, there was nothing she could do for me. But there was a lot I could do for myself. If there's one thing my months of playing this game have taught me it's that I can start over at any time. I can start my day over, I can start my mood over, I can start my week or month or morning or moment over. I put down my computer about an hour ago and I got up and I walked the 200 feet to the ocean. I played with my baby and splashed in the water with my husband and my sister-in-law. I took a jog down the beach and did a little yoga on some rocks perched out over the water. And then I sat down and meditated for 5 minutes before I jogged back to play with my baby some more.

I was on the beach for about an hour. And EVERYTHING shifted. I got my sanity back. I came back to the house and I ate a plum and then I sat back down to write, feeling like a *wholly different human being.*

Amazingly, I have tools now. I know exactly what I need to do to feel better. I need to eat well. I need to sleep enough, even when it feels impossible. I need to play and I need to drink water and get a little exercise and maybe sit still and contemplate something larger than myself for a few minutes. I need a little balance.

If you are reading this before playing the game, then please come back and read it again in four weeks. My hope is that you will experience what I'm describing by playing. My hope is that you will, once the game is over, go back to your regular life and apply the principles you've learned and when you forget to apply them and start to feel like crap again, you'll remember in short order and apply them again. My hope is also that you'll play again whenever you want to or need to—but that in between games, you'll utilize the tools you've picked up and draw on the community you've built by playing.

Remember, this isn't just a diet. A diet has a start and a finish and then sends you back to your regular life to fall apart until you're ready to start the diet again. This game is designed to teach you and your friends and family a way of life that you can keep on living together long after the trash-talk has subsided and the prizes have been collected.

> *I loved the game! The last week of it, I pretty much had it down as a habit. When it was over, I made the effortless decision to continue with this new lifestyle. I was in good health and had good habits before the game. But the game gave me great health and a great structure to live by.*
>
> —Sarah, 26

Once the game is over, take a week off and see what you can carry into your game-free life. My guess is you'll keep exercising a little and if you're like me, your body will now crave the extra water and the fresh fruits and veggies. See what you can do while you're not competing and then, when you want to, whether it's after a week or a month, PLAY AGAIN. I have lost forty pounds playing this game and I'm still going. And yes, in between games, I occasionally gain a pound or two back, but much more often, I continue to lose or I hold my weight steady—despite tight deadlines and long work hours; despite an addictive personality and a genetic predisposition for obesity and happy laziness. If I can do this, you can do this. You can change your body. You can change your life. And when you slide back into old habits, you can start over again. One game, one day, one hour, one point at a time.

## • • • A Tip from Az • • •

No matter how far you've come on your journey toward the healthiest possible you, stop now and acknowledge yourself. For just a moment, take note of your success, take note of your accomplishments, take note of all your hard work. Maybe you've met your fitness goals, maybe you still have miles to go—but you've taken a big step forward by embarking on this game and I really want you to take the time to appreciate your own efforts. Most of us beat ourselves up for a thousand reasons every day. Let's balance that a little by giving ourselves credit for how far we've come.

## Frequently Asked Questions

Q: My team is training for a marathon. Can we play one game for seven weeks instead of four?

A: Absolutely! The first game we ever played lasted nine weeks. That said, we were a little sick of it at the end of nine weeks. By limiting it to four weeks, we've found that we are always eager to start again. But if you're using it to train for a marathon, I say go go go!

Q: I want to keep eating and exercising the same way but I don't want to play another game with a team. Any suggestions as to how to stay motivated?

A: Notice how much better you feel physically and emotionally when you are treating your body well. And if that doesn't work, reread Chapter 4, Playing by Yourself. You might find some tidbits in there to keep you going.

Q:   None of my clothes fit now but I'm afraid to throw them away in case I get fat again. What should I do?

A:   GIVE THEM AWAY! Bundle up every item that is too big and drive it to a homeless shelter (or a local church or Goodwill). This is (a) a great good deed and (b) makes getting fat again a way less appealing option because when you start to gain weight you will have nothing to wear! The first time you start thinking about going out and buying bigger clothes, you will KNOW it's time to play again!

Q:   Now that I've lost all this weight, I get a lot more attention from guys. It makes me a little uncomfortable because I'm so used to being the fat girl. When I get uncomfortable, I start to feel the need to hide behind my weight again, but I don't want to gain it all back. Any suggestions??

A:   Get a good therapist. I mean it. Good therapy blew my life wide open. I can't recommend it highly enough.

## GET A PEN!

In the following spaces, write at least three things you accomplished by playing this game. Then write three more things you'd like to accomplish when next you play.

_____

_____

_____

_____

_____

_____

_____

_____

## Jana Harper, *15 pounds lost*

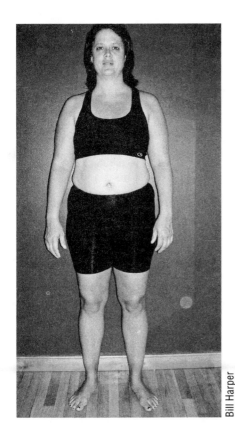
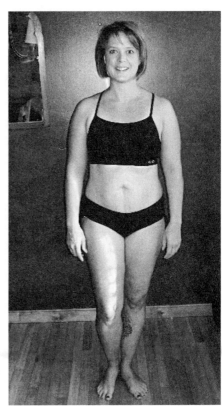

Bill Harper

Bill Harper

When my son was two, I could no longer claim that the extra pounds I was carrying were "baby fat." I embarked on losing weight. I did a twelve-week program to get the ball rolling but had a hard time staying motivated. When Krista said she and Aaron were starting a game to lose weight I thought, "What do I have to lose?" I'm competitive and love having set "rules" to work within. I did however believe they were crazy when they told me I had to get seven hours of sleep a night. Crazy! I had been getting along just fine on five to six hours, thank you very much. But I wanted to win so I figured I would give it a go.

I not only lost weight and got into better shape, I was having fewer memory issues, my mood was better, and I had loads and loads of patience for my children. The latter was so profound for me. Five to six hours of sleep had not afforded me much patience and, in hindsight, I realize my kids and husband suffered as well. Now I'm rested, eating better, and in the best shape I have been in for twenty years! All while beating my friends at a game (except in the end, the girls lost). But it was a win for ME! I love how this game has evolved and I am still motivated to play and pursue increasing my health for myself and my children. I am doing things today that I did not think possible. All in all I have lost nearly thirty pounds (the last fifteen by playing the game), but, more important, I have found a sense of joy and play again. I love new challenges, I love showing my kids how fun being active can be, and I love being able to keep up with them! And now, even if I'm not playing a game, I have the tools to take better care of myself. I know and my body really knows when I am not treating it right. Play! What do you have to lose?

Jana, 40

# Chapter 18

# PEP TALK

## (Or, GAME ON!)

Finish every day and be done with it.
You have done what you could;
some absurdities crept in;
forget them as soon as you can.
Tomorrow is a new day;
you shall begin it serenely
and with too high a spirit to be
encumbered with your old nonsense.

—*Ralph Waldo Emerson*

**You are not** just your body. But your body and its state of health inform your well-being—your thoughts, your heart, your spirit. What you are doing by playing this game is monumental. What you are saying to the world by playing this game is, *I rock. I just fucking rock. I am not a victim of anything or anyone. I am certainly not a victim of my cellulite. I can effect change in the world and I'm going to start with my physical health. So there, fuckers!*

If you are not as big on the F word as I am, feel free to modify the above statement according to your taste—but know that the spirit is right. Don't come to this game feeling like you have to play because you're fat and gross. Come to this game knowing that you are playing because you are alive and you are vibrant and you are capable and you want to live your fullest, happiest, healthiest life.

Don't come to this game because you are defeated. Come because you are determined and inspired. Come because despite how you may feel, feelings are not facts. The facts are (or I hope they are) that you are healthy and physically able to take this on. The facts are that no matter what your experience has been in the past, you have the power to change your experiences in the future.

If you put words in your head and in your heart like, "I'm playing this game because I'm so fat and gross," you might make your points but you're not gonna have nearly as good a time doing it. Life is too short for that shit. You wouldn't take it from a friend so don't take it from yourself. Replace the negative thoughts with *the truth*. The truth is that if you *take healthy actions* one meal, one hour, one day at a time, your body and your heart and your mind and your life will transform. It just will.

When I catch myself feeling sorry for myself or feeling bad about my body, I put on some happy music and jump around my bedroom, and OUT LOUD I give thanks that I *can* jump. Try it. (And if you have a kid, do it with your kid—it's even better. And if you have a dog, your dog will love it!)

If a couple of songs' worth of that doesn't work, call in sick (because you are sick, you are soul-sick) and head down to your local soup kitchen and be of service to the homeless for the day. Or go to the library and teach an illiterate adult to read. I promise you, you will leave with a new perspective on the extra calories you consumed or the coworker who was mean to you or whatever kind of bad day you couldn't shake.

If you feel as if you might quit, remind yourself why you took this on. Is it because of your health? Your waistline? Your self-esteem? All three? Remind yourself and then recommit.

You are kick-ass. You know it, and I know it. And if you don't know it, read this quotation from Marianne Williamson and then come talk to me.

*Our deepest fear is not that we are inadequate. Our deepest fear is that we are powerful beyond measure. It is our light, not our darkness, that most frightens us. We ask ourselves, who am I to be brilliant, gorgeous, talented, fabulous? Actually, who are you not to be? You are a child of God. Your playing small doesn't serve the world. There's nothing enlightened about shrinking so that other people won't feel insecure around you. We are all meant to shine, as children do. We were born to make manifest the glory of God that is within us. It's not just in some of us; it's in everyone. And as we let our own light shine, we unconsciously give other people permission to do the same. As we're liberated from our own fear, our presence automatically liberates others.*

Play the game. Play all out. Bring your whole self. Bring your fears and bring your joys and bring your competitive spirit and bring your trash-talk. Bring it. You know you want to. GAME ON!

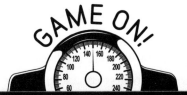

| Week 1 Weight Chart | |
|---|---|
| Starting Weight | |
| Goal Weight | |
| End Weight | |

## SCOREBOARD week 1

| | Mon | Tues | Wed | Thurs | Fri | Sat | Sun | TOTAL POINTS |
|---|---|---|---|---|---|---|---|---|
| **Points Scored:** | | | | | | | | |
| MEALS (6 points per meal) | | | | | | | | |
| | | | | | | | | |
| | | | | | | | | |
| | | | | | | | | |
| | | | | | | | | |
| | | | | | | | | |
| daily total | | | | | | | | /210 |
| EXERCISE (20 points) | | | | | | | | |
| | | | | | | | | /140 |
| SLEEP (15 points) | | | | | | | | |
| 7+ hours | | | | | | | | /105 |
| WATER (10 points) | | | | | | | | |
| 3 liters | | | | | | | | /70 |
| NEW HABIT (10 points) | | | | | | | | |
| | | | | | | | | /70 |
| OLD HABIT (10 points) | | | | | | | | |
| | | | | | | | | /70 |
| COMMUNICATION (5 points) | | | | | | | | |
| | | | | | | | | /35 |
| **Penalties:** | | | | | | | | |
| SCALE PENALTY (Deduct 1 point per penalty) | | | | | | | | |
| | | | | | | | | - |
| SNACKING PENALTY (Deduct 10 points per penalty) | | | | | | | | |
| | | | | | | | | - |
| COLLUSION PENALTY (Deduct 20 points per penalty) | | | | | | | | |
| | | | | | | | | - |
| ALCOHOL (Deduct 25 points per penalty) | | | | | | | | |
| | | | | | | | | - |
| CHANGE YOUR HABIT (deduct 50 points) | | | | | | | | |
| | | | | | | | | - |
| **SUB TOTAL FOR THE WEEK** | | | | | | | | /700 |
| **Bonus Points:** | | | | | | | | |
| **Add 20%** of total points earned if you reached your fitness or weightloss goal (lost 1% of your starting weight for the week) | | | | | | | | |
| **Add 10 points** for reporting your score to your team scorekeeper on time. | | | | | | | | |
| **TOTAL POINTS FOR THE WEEK** | | | | | | | | /850 |

Note: Give yourself full points for your day off and your meal off.

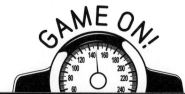

| Week 2 Weight Chart | |
|---|---|
| Starting Weight | |
| Goal Weight | |
| End Weight | |

## SCOREBOARD week 2

| | Mon | Tues | Wed | Thurs | Fri | Sat | Sun | TOTAL POINTS |
|---|---|---|---|---|---|---|---|---|
| **Points Scored:** | | | | | | | | |
| MEALS (6 points per meal) | | | | | | | | |
| | | | | | | | | |
| | | | | | | | | |
| | | | | | | | | |
| | | | | | | | | |
| daily total | | | | | | | | /210 |
| EXERCISE (20 points) | | | | | | | | |
| | | | | | | | | /140 |
| SLEEP (15 points) | | | | | | | | |
| 7+ hours | | | | | | | | /105 |
| WATER (10 points) | | | | | | | | |
| 3 liters | | | | | | | | /70 |
| NEW HABIT (10 points) | | | | | | | | |
| | | | | | | | | /70 |
| OLD HABIT (10 points) | | | | | | | | |
| | | | | | | | | /70 |
| COMMUNICATION (5 points) | | | | | | | | |
| | | | | | | | | /35 |
| **Penalties:** | | | | | | | | |
| SCALE PENALTY (Deduct 1 point per penalty) | | | | | | | | |
| | | | | | | | | - |
| SNACKING PENALTY (Deduct 10 points per penalty) | | | | | | | | |
| | | | | | | | | - |
| COLLUSION PENALTY (Deduct 20 points per penality) | | | | | | | | |
| | | | | | | | | - |
| ALCOHOL (Deduct 25 points per penalty) | | | | | | | | |
| | | | | | | | | - |
| CHANGE YOUR HABIT (deduct 50 points) | | | | | | | | |
| | | | | | | | | - |
| **SUB TOTAL FOR THE WEEK** | | | | | | | | /700 |
| **Bonus Points:** | | | | | | | | |
| **Add 20%** of total points earned if you reached your fitness or weightloss goal (lost 1% of your starting weight for the week) | | | | | | | | |
| **Add 10 points** for reporting your score to your team scorekeeper on time. | | | | | | | | |
| **TOTAL POINTS FOR THE WEEK** | | | | | | | | /850 |

Note: Give yourself full points for your day off and your meal off.

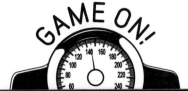

| Week 3 Weight Chart | |
|---|---|
| Starting Weight | |
| Goal Weight | |
| End Weight | |

## SCOREBOARD  week 3

| | Mon | Tues | Wed | Thurs | Fri | Sat | Sun | TOTAL POINTS |
|---|---|---|---|---|---|---|---|---|
| **Points Scored:** | | | | | | | | |
| MEALS (6 points per meal) | | | | | | | | |
| | | | | | | | | |
| | | | | | | | | |
| | | | | | | | | |
| | | | | | | | | |
| daily total | | | | | | | | /210 |
| EXERCISE (20 points) | | | | | | | | |
| | | | | | | | | /140 |
| SLEEP (15 points) | | | | | | | | |
| 7+ hours | | | | | | | | /105 |
| WATER (10 points) | | | | | | | | |
| 3 liters | | | | | | | | /70 |
| NEW HABIT (10 points) | | | | | | | | |
| | | | | | | | | /70 |
| OLD HABIT (10 points) | | | | | | | | |
| | | | | | | | | /70 |
| COMMUNICATION (5 points) | | | | | | | | |
| | | | | | | | | /35 |
| **Penalties:** | | | | | | | | |
| SCALE PENALTY (Deduct 1 point per penalty) | | | | | | | | |
| | | | | | | | | - |
| SNACKING PENALTY (Deduct 10 points per penalty) | | | | | | | | |
| | | | | | | | | - |
| COLLUSION PENALTY (Deduct 20 points per penalty) | | | | | | | | |
| | | | | | | | | - |
| ALCOHOL (Deduct 25 points per penalty) | | | | | | | | |
| | | | | | | | | - |
| CHANGE YOUR HABIT (deduct 50 points) | | | | | | | | |
| | | | | | | | | - |
| **SUB TOTAL FOR THE WEEK** | | | | | | | | /700 |
| **Bonus Points:** | | | | | | | | |
| **Add 20%** of total points earned if you reached your fitness or weightloss goal (lost 1% of your starting weight for the week) | | | | | | | | |
| **Add 10 points** for reporting your score to your team scorekeeper on time. | | | | | | | | |
| **TOTAL POINTS FOR THE WEEK** | | | | | | | | /850 |

Note: Give yourself full points for your day off and your meal off.

| Week 4 Weight Chart | |
|---|---|
| Starting Weight | |
| Goal Weight | |
| End Weight | |

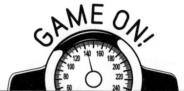

## SCOREBOARD week 4

| | Mon | Tues | Wed | Thurs | Fri | Sat | Sun | TOTAL POINTS |
|---|---|---|---|---|---|---|---|---|
| **Points Scored:** | | | | | | | | |
| MEALS (6 points per meal) | | | | | | | | |
| | | | | | | | | |
| | | | | | | | | |
| | | | | | | | | |
| | | | | | | | | |
| | | | | | | | | |
| daily total | | | | | | | | /210 |
| EXERCISE (20 points) | | | | | | | | |
| | | | | | | | | /140 |
| SLEEP (15 points) | | | | | | | | |
| 7+ hours | | | | | | | | /105 |
| WATER (10 points) | | | | | | | | |
| 3 liters | | | | | | | | /70 |
| NEW HABIT (10 points) | | | | | | | | |
| | | | | | | | | /70 |
| OLD HABIT (10 points) | | | | | | | | |
| | | | | | | | | /70 |
| COMMUNICATION (5 points) | | | | | | | | |
| | | | | | | | | /35 |
| **Penalties:** | | | | | | | | |
| SCALE PENALTY (Deduct 1 point per penalty) | | | | | | | | |
| | | | | | | | - | |
| SNACKING PENALTY (Deduct 10 points per penalty) | | | | | | | | |
| | | | | | | | - | |
| COLLUSION PENALTY (Deduct 20 points per penality) | | | | | | | | |
| | | | | | | | - | |
| ALCOHOL (Deduct 25 points per penalty) | | | | | | | | |
| | | | | | | | - | |
| CHANGE YOUR HABIT (deduct 50 points) | | | | | | | | |
| | | | | | | | - | |
| **SUB TOTAL FOR THE WEEK** | | | | | | | | /700 |
| **Bonus Points:** | | | | | | | | |
| **Add 20%** of total points earned if you reached your fitness or weightloss goal (lost 1% of your starting weight for the week) | | | | | | | | |
| **Add 10 points** for reporting your score to your team scorekeeper on time. | | | | | | | | |
| **TOTAL POINTS FOR THE WEEK** | | | | | | | | /850 |

Note: Give yourself full points for your day off and your meal off.

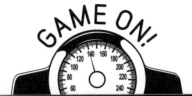

| Final Weight Chart: | |
|---|---|
| Starting Weight | |
| Goal Weight | |
| End Weight | |

## SCOREBOARD TOTAL

| WEEK 1 | | TOTAL POINTS | /850 |
|---|---|---|---|
| WEEK 2 | | TOTAL POINTS | /850 |
| WEEK 3 | | TOTAL POINTS | /850 |
| WEEK 4 | | TOTAL POINTS | /850 |
| | | TOTAL POINTS FOR THE GAME | /3400 |

# Contributors

**Heide Banks**, who has an MA in spiritual psychology, is a master in helping individuals to release blocks and unleash their true self-expression, the ultimate key to success in all areas of our lives. Her insightful work in relationships, career, and health has made her a fixture in the national media with regular appearances on such shows as *The Oprah Winfrey Show*, CNN, *Entertainment Tonight*, and *The Tyra Banks Show*. In addition, Heide serves as the executive director of the Center for Partnership Studies and is its representative to the United Nations. For media and more information about her coaching services, Heide can be reached at HeideBanks.com.

**Dr. Michael Bernard Beckwith** is the founder of the Agape International Spiritual Center, located in Los Angeles, California. Agape is a trans-religious community that today counts a membership of thousands locally, and hundreds of thousands of worldwide friends, as well as regional and international affiliates. Dr. Beckwith is a sought after meditation teacher, and facilitates conferences and seminars on the Life Visioning Process, which he originated. He is the author of *Spiritual Liberation: Fulfilling Your Soul's Potential*, *Inspirations of the Heart*, *Forty Day Mind Fast-Soul Feast*, and *A Manifesto of Peace*. He has appeared on *The Oprah Winfrey Show*, *Larry King Live*, and is a featured teacher in the book and film *The Secret*. He is also featured in the following films: *The Moses Code*, *Pass It On*, and *Living Luminaries*. For more information visit www.agapelive.com.

**Jen Bloom** brings her practical out-of-the-studio style of yoga right to where you need it: the stressful situations of everyday life. Her revolutionary *Yoga in the Car* CD has been featured on ABC *Boston Chronicle*, online by *Yoga Journal*, and received Best in Show for the CA Gift Show by New Age Retailer. *Yoga on the Plane* and *Yoga for the Armchair* are on their way! A cancer survivor, Jen works with private clients to bring the gentler aspects of yoga into their healing process. She teaches workshops throughout L.A. To book a session or take a class, please visit www.yogablooms.com.

**Jennifer Burton,** MFT, CEAT, is a Los Angeles–based therapist specializing in trauma and other life issues. Along with talk therapy, Jennifer practices Expressive Arts Therapy and is certified in EMDR and Integrated Somatic Therapy. For a consultation or more information go to www.jenniferburtonmft.com or call 310-630-4300.

**Zoanne Clack,** MD, MPH, FACEP is a writer/producer/medical consultant on ABC's hit television show *Grey's Anatomy* and a practicing emergency physician. She is a true believer in the power of the entertainment field to influence social norms and has become dedicated to promoting social and behavioral change through the dissemination of public health issues in the media. Her holistic approach includes disease prevention and healthy lifestyles as well as traditional treatment options.

**Laurie Sansone Ferguson,** CAES, a language and literacy specialist, has served for two decades as an instructor, teacher educator, and mentor, providing language and literacy instruction and pedagogical professional development in Europe, Asia, South America, and the United States.

**Michelle Fiordaliso,** MSW, CNC, is a writer, psychotherapist, and nutritional consultant. She earned both her undergraduate degree and her master's degree in clinical social work from New York University and has counseled individuals and couples for the past fifteen years. As the clinical director of ShrinkYourself.com she has helped thousands of people overcome lifelong struggles with bingeing, food addiction, and emotional eating. Michelle is the 2008 recipient of the PEN USA Community Access Scholarship for writing, a 2007 finalist for The Sherwood Award and has a relationship book coming out in April 2009, which is being published by Sourcebooks. A regular blogger on sites such as The Huffington Post, eHarmony.com, and TheHotMom'sClub.com, she lives in Los Angeles with her son. For more information: www.michellefiordaliso.com.

**Leo Galland,** M.D., has received international recognition as a leader in the field of nutritional medicine over the past twenty-five years. A board-certified internist with a practice in New York City, Dr. Galland is the author of numerous scientific articles and textbook chapters and three highly acclaimed books, *Superimmunity for Kids*, *Power Healing*, and *The Fat Resistance Diet*.

*Jessica Jennings* started practicing yoga in 1997 for chronic pain in her neck, and long after the pain was gone she continued to enjoy how good yoga made her feel. She has a master of science degree in kinesiology with a focus on rehab exercise, is a certified fitness instructor, and a certified Anusara yoga teacher. Jessica loves to share the gifts of yoga with people of every fitness level, age, and size, and specializes in therapeutics for injuries and pain, as well as yoga for pregnancy. For personalized yoga training or to find classes in the Los Angeles area, go to www.yogagroundwork.com.

*David L. Katz* MD, MPH, FACPM, FACP, is a board-certified specialist in both internal medicine and preventive medicine/public health. He is an Associate Professor (adjunct) at the Yale School of Public Health, and Director of Yale University's Prevention Research Center. He has authored eleven books to date, including two editions of a nutrition textbook for health care professionals. He is the founder and director of the Integrative Medicine Center at Griffin Hospital in Derby, Conneticut, a facility with a unique and nationally recognized model of evidence-based holistic care; and the founder and president of the nonprofit Turn the Tide Foundation, devoted to reversing trends in obesity and related chronic disease.

*Jennifer L. Kelman*, LMSW, is a clinical social worker and weight loss coach practicing in New York and Florida. She founded Weight Loss Coaching and Consulting, LLC, which provides individualized care to weight-loss clients. Jennifer has lectured extensively around the country on various topics including body image, eating disorders, and weight loss. For a consult, call 561-368-1741.

*Doug Kraft* has been training Hollywood for over ten years with a strong background in core and functional training. For your own personal training consultation go to www.dougkraft.com.

*Dr. Joseph Mercola* is the founder of Dr. Mercola's Natural Health Center, near Chicago, Illinois. His Web site, www.Mercola.com, is the most popular natural health Web site in the world.

*Sue Molnar* has been teaching spinning in Los Angeles and New York for over ten years. For great playlists, workout tunes, and tips for your fitness regimen, check out www.SuesTrax.com.

**Deepak Ramapriyan** is a Los Angeles–based music instructor, record producer, and mathematician and the Director of *FUNdamentals of Music and Movement*, a San Fernando Valley Franchise. He is also the creator of the rock band The B.O.L.T. (Breath of Life Tribe). For more information go to www.theotherdeepak.com.

**Fay Wolf** brings order and peace of mind to the Los Angeles area. She is an active member of the National Association of Professional Organizers (NAPO) and has been featured on *Apartment Therapy* and in *Los Angeles Confidential* magazine. Her celebrity client list includes Rachael Leigh Cook, Emily and Zooey Deschanel, Alyson Hannigan, and Michael Urie. For a personal consult please go to www.neworderorganizing.com.

# Acknowledgments

We are so deeply grateful to everyone who helped us along the crazy path of first time authors. Without your help, love, and support this book would not exist. You know it, we know it, and now we'd like the world to know it.

### From Krista

Thank you from the bottom of my heart to . . .

My Kevy, who waited so patiently while I disappeared into these pages for months.

Andy Elkin, who so kindly did not freak out when I told him I was writing a book instead of a TV show.

My mom, Aysha, who inspires me every day to keep questioning the medical establishment and to keep seeking natural and organic foods and medicines.

Sue, Mary, Katy, and Emily, who supported this idea with wild enthusiasm and saved me this year, one Sunday at a time.

Natalia, Gail, Carol, and Toia, who, along with Kimberly, brought me here.

My sister Kaili, who read the first draft and cheered me on, and my sister Sydni, who babysat a lot so I could write. My sister Jenn, who is actually a shrink and is still so loving and patient when I try to pretend I'm one too. My brother Tony, who always makes me laugh.

My stepdad, John, who lovingly snapped my fat "before" photos even though he thought he was just taking my picture.

My stepmom, Saba, who says "you're so wonderful" even when I'm not feeling wonderful, and my dad, Bob Verne, whom we both still miss terribly.

Beverly, Bob, and Kristin Maynard, and all my in-laws who so kindly understood when I showed up for an hour and a half of a weeklong family vacation.

Star Michael and Blanca Hernandez, who take such wonderful care of us every day and overtime.

Peter Paige, who is my one and only Peter Paige.

Shonda, Hammer, Tony, Joan, Debora, Allan, Jenna, Zoanne, Stacy, Bill, Pete, Austin, Elizabeth, Moira, Sonay, and Meg, the *Grey's Anatomy* tribe, who loved and mocked me and helped me through a whole new onslaught of book-related neuroses (and who make me laugh really hard every day).

Every teacher I've ever had.

And Az, who is so truly generous and who was kind enough to help me get way less fat.

## From Az

Thank you from the bottom of my heart to . . .

Mum, whose enthusiasm for anything I take on is unparalleled and whose hugs make the world melt away.

Mike, who took Jazzie and me on as his own and made us laugh until we cried.

Jazzie and Ted—my greatest pastime growing up was to make Jazzie laugh—thanks for making it so easy, and thanks to Ted for bringing such joy to one of the greatest people on this earth.

Krista Vernoff, who continually inspires me.

Adam and Andie Skovron, who always see me as my greatest self and lovingly let me know when I'm being less than who I can be.

The Collins tribe: Greg, Mandy, Kristen, Griffin, Jasper, and Charlie, who made "Coming to America" the easiest decision.

Phil and Woody, who make being an adult bearable by always letting me play like a kid.

My aunties, Meg and Gila; growing up with the Nelson ladies was one of my greatest joys. Thanks for showing me so much life.

My American family, who so generously adopted me: Jesse, Jojo, Kate, Kristen, Sammy, Peter, Brooke and Tom, Jana and Billy, Krista and Kevin, Mandi and Greg, Michaela and Casey. It's been an absolute cracker!

Finally, to the thousands of people who have inspired me throughout my life, some I knew personally, some I never met. I apologize that I didn't thank you in the moment, and I promise that I'll take that on as my "New Habit" for it is these acts of inspiration that make the world such a magical place to live. Thank You!

## From Both of Us

Thank you so, so, so much . . .

Lisa Sharkey and Amy Kaplan, our incredible editors, who simply rock in every possible way.

Lisa Shotland, Rich Green, and Jamie Mandelbaum, who know a lot of stuff we don't and helped enormously.

The wonderful Mandy Collins, who introduced us.

Stacy McKee, Brooke Blanchard, Greg Collins, and Andie Skouron, for their artistry, speed, experience, and generosity.

Every friend and friend of a friend who played the game with passion and offered us their time, feedback, wisdom, questions, photos, recipes, and quotes.

All of our expert contributors, who so generously shared their wisdom and counsel on the pages of this book.

Blain Bovee, our brilliant astrologer, who said "write the book!!!" (www .BoveeAstrology.com)

Mickey, Jana, Kevin, and Anselm—the original players. We would like to note that the girls have still not paid up on those show tickets.

And a very special thanks to Tammy Duffy, who researched and read tirelessly for months and really, truly made this book possible.